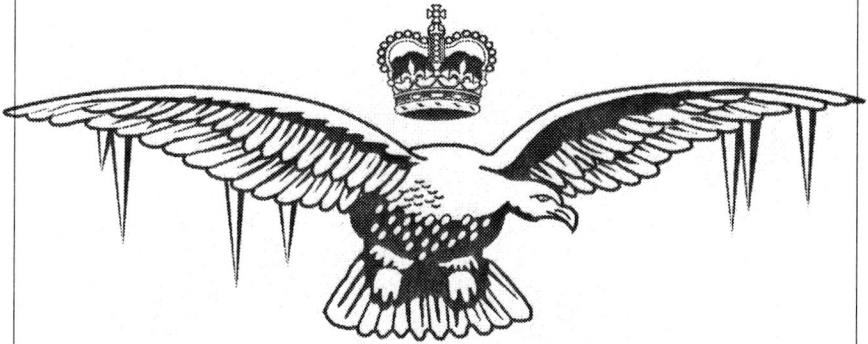

ICE ON MY WINGS

SQUADRON LEADER JOHN FARRON MBE

Bloomington, IN   authorHOUSE®   Milton Keynes, UK

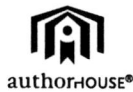

AuthorHouse™
1663 Liberty Drive, Suite 200
Bloomington, IN 47403
www.authorhouse.com
Phone: 1-800-839-8640

AuthorHouse™ UK Ltd.
500 Avebury Boulevard
Central Milton Keynes, MK9 2BE
www.authorhouse.co.uk
Phone: 08001974150

First published by AuthorHouse 3/30/2007

ISBN: 978-1-4259-8146-4 (sc)

Printed in the United States of America
Bloomington, Indiana

This book is printed on acid-free paper.

INTRODUCTION

This book is about entering, surviving and discovering the truths and the untruths of suffering deepest depression and the vicissitudes of life so far.

It is a humorous, some times heart-breaking and yet a heart-warming story of mind over matter, of medical miracles and life-changing events told by a pilot as viewed from his cockpit of life. Having no medical training, the author describes the symptoms in aeronautical terms which are analogous to the conditions directly observed during this serious illness.

Depression has overtaken heart disease as the world's No. 1 illness. He knows. He survived both. Little is known about depression. There is much theory. Few facts emerge from direct experience as the few survive to tell their true story of the uncontrolled spin of this deadly unstable condition we call depression.

It has been estimated that over 300 million people in the world today suffer from it. Depression was first named as a condition about 2,400 years ago by the ancient Greek doctor Hippocrates, who called it 'melancholia'.

This is a story of how one goes into deep depression, some of the causes, and how to survive it, what it is like in it and how to recover from it and some tips on how to avoid re entry. The story is told by someone who observed the whole process from darkness to light, from life to death and back again.

This is not an autobiography but periods of the life have been described in the context in which the depression has appeared to illustrate how it is related to the individual nature of the person it has diseased. It thereby helps both the author and the reader to come to a measure of understanding of the phenomenon Winston Churchill called 'the Black Dog' and Alexander the Great called 'the Great Melancholy'

This book is dedicated to the author's family, friends, his professional and flying colleagues and Dr. Pradip Patel who helped him to survive the stormiest flight of his life.

The expression 'Ice on your wings' is part of the friendly but competitive world of banter often used amongst military aircrew in meeting the challenges of their profession, remaining in high spirits and above all maintaining their sense of humour about the risky business of living and flying. In reality, it is of course, a very dangerous aerodynamic condition.

John Farron is a Squadron Leader in the Royal Air Force Volunteer Reserve (Training Branch). He is a Qualified Gliding Instructor, has a Private Pilots Licence and holds an appointment as Special Projects Officer for Headquarters Air Cadets, Royal Air Force College, Cranwell. He was appointed MBE by the Queen in 2001, is a 'Fellow of the Royal Aeronautical Society' and runs his own Business Development Consultancy.

FOREWORD

BY DR. PRADIP PATEL – CONSULTANT PSYCHIATRIST

I thoroughly enjoyed reading the excellent account of your journey through depression. I enjoyed the mixture of humour and serious thought. I found the account of your hospital admission for depression thought provoking. The 'fictional' but real characters were humorous! It made me think about the power of 'sectioning' and how easily this could be used in a harmful way if there are not enough safeguards. I think your view of what happened is important for professionals to hear about and bear in mind when making decisions about taking another person's liberty away. I would not want you to change this account in any way as it contains some important issues that need further thought by services and patients.

The remarkable support you have had from friends and family is recorded well. I had a hearty laugh at the section entitled 'Is thinking destroying your life'. This is so true. One could say that both depression and anxiety are good examples of illnesses where too much 'negative' and 'catastrophic' thinking leads to harm and stops recovery. I found the account of your childhood in Preston and Darwen interesting. The manuscript has helped me understand much more about the 'person' you are and the sheer determination and the 'will' to survive that you so evidently have. I think your remarkable story of survival would give hope to other sufferers of depression. In chapter eight, I like the emphasis on what depression is and what it is not. It is a serious illness and it is survivable, as you have shown. You have also shown how it can make one stronger and survive further major stresses without becoming depressed again.

I have learnt from you the importance of helping a sufferer understand that depression is separate from the person who is ill. Depression makes one forget who one is and I like the idea of family and friends 'holding', 'remembering' this person for the sufferer, till they begin to recover. The letters spelling DEPRESSION have so much in them as you have shown with both wit and humour. Your philosophical views are interesting as are your aeronautical 'models'. Your account has made me realise how important family and friends are and how little 'professionals' can do if one doesn't have such support. I am truly glad that you have recovered and in the process have hopefully become more 'self-aware' and thus finally fulfilled your true potential. I hope the self-confidence you feel now will never again be taken away by depression.

When you gave me the manuscript you had asked me not to hesitate to make critical comments if I had any. I don't really have any. I was delighted to see how well you were able to describe the 'stormiest flight of your life'. I think your experience of what helped you make the final breakthrough would be of great value to other sufferers of depression. As you say for the sufferer ultimately there is a stark black and white choice i.e. 'live or die'. You chose to live. I presume the support of your friends and family was crucial in choosing to live. Your account has also made me think more about models professionals could use to explain what happens during depression. There is the well known psychological model called Beck's 'negative cognitive triad' that helps one understand how thinking and judgement can be skewed by depression and the links between negative thoughts and low mood and how the former maintain low mood as a vicious circle that is difficult to break out of.

REVIEW

BY GROUP CAPTAIN W M N CROSS OBE

I felt very privileged when John Farron invited me to review his book, particularly as I have not experience the downs and ups which John captures so well. I have known John for some 13 years during my tenure as Chief of Staff of the Air Cadet Organisation. Over that time I have seen at first hand the enormous commitment in several capacities which John has voluntarily made to the Organisation and which has had a significant impact.

His book is deeply personal. One is drawn into the struggle he went through as his affliction took its grip, but, because of the nature of the man, also the effort he had to make to accept that he had a problem and then to express publicly the emotions and experiences he found himself faced with. He vividly describes his descent into a personal dungeon using analogies drawn from his piloting experience.

He goes on to use flying analogies to provide a reference point for achieving some sort of stability, then hope, and finally to emerge into light again. Just as striking is the military ethos and personal discipline he had developed during his time as a volunteer officer which helped him rebuild a framework to his life offering him a straw to hang onto and to eventually recover.

This is well expressed in the later passages when he describes that same ethos which he found in his friends and old gliding colleagues who by guile, and above all 'looking out for one's mate', restored his confidence to the extent that he was able to take up once again the strands of life which had meant so much to him. Above all his family, despite all the difficulties, never abandoned him; their constancy provided another essential platform for his survival and recovery.

This is an intense and brave book which explores an aspect of the human lot which many people so affected are unwilling to, or fail to, face up to. Hopefully for those it will help to open seemingly impenetrable doors.

CONTENTS

1 ELLEN STREET

Popular legend has it that I was born during an air raid at 172 Ellen street, Preston on 25th January 1941. Popular that is, with my mother Marcella and my paternal grandmother Mary Ellen who used to tell me the street was named after her.

Apparently they wrapped me in swaddling clothes and hid me under the bed in a Moses basket until the Jerry's had gone and just in case the neighbours called in to see what was causing all the noise, as they could not hear the bombing over my yelling.

So began a lifetime of hidden feelings of inferiority, sought but not found, heard but not seen, out of mind, out of sight, swept under the bed, the carpet you know that sort of thing. Moses basket eh! What were they planning next?

It seems that the German bombers where looking for Dick Kerr's aircraft factory and Preston Docks just down the road from Mary Ellen's street and a stick of bombs fell in nearby Moor Park creating even more tank trap holes to stop them landing their Mercedes Tiger tanks or even gliders! More of these later.

But for me the war was over as I dozed off, still under the bed, watching the silver fish scuttle over the emerald green tiles on the front room parlour fireplace as the bright warm glow of the coal fire settled down for the long dark mid winters night.

Ellen street, not quite Penny Lane , more of an Eleanor Rigby street with its respectable well built terraced houses and a Mrs Penswick next door to watch the world for you. But for me it was my entire universe as I often viewed it from my Silver Cross,

1

lower middle class pram, parked by my mum under grandma's front parlour window directly opposite Titteringtons' saw mill on the other side of the street. I will never forget that glorious sweet apple cider smell of freshly sawn planks of virgin soft wood and the whine of the insatiable ripping saw.

These were magical days when I was blissfully happy in the absolute knowledge and the joy of just being in the present moment and the truly natural state of mind which is every child's birthright.

Yes I can recall it as though it was yesterday; indeed all my troubles were so faraway and not for sometime yet was I to forget the beautiful feeling of the natural bliss of (as Pooh Bear would say) just being!

But eventually the game of life would inexorably begin and I would by nature be compelled to play the process of forgetting who I really am and adopt this false persona which the eastern philosophical traditions call Ahankara and the westerner's call Ego.

Meanwhile back in Ellen Street I had graduated from the regal peaceful palace of the pram and had come down to the shop floor of life; the concrete surface of the road outside 172 where I had made an amazing scientific discovery called tar! This was so enthralling that I began to practise my new found skill of forgetting. In those days mothers could let their children play on the street unattended for hours, and my mother often did. As I discovered, she also had learnt to forget - me!

This was now my total world, my universe, my all. The smell, the feel, the glistening sight of this elastic substance – tar, tar, glorious tar! So there I lay in the middle of the street with my fingers and nose in it, my whole being in it, oblivious to anything else in or on this empty street which led to the busy main Garstang Road along which armies marched, trucks rumbled and tanks trundled off to war. But I had my tar.

But then this was war time and there were no private cars, no gas squandering 4x4's, Chelsea tractors with extra bull bars to run down any working class insurrection, just a solitary, tar covered, lower middle class forgotten two year old in the middle of an empty street. No school run, no need for yellow lines except for those indicating EWS, emergency water supply, daubed like an early form of official graffiti on every street corner ready for the next incendiary bomb or chip pan fire. Just think if one fell on that golden mountain of sweet smelling sawdust in Titterington's yard, a fire bomb that is, would EWS cope?

Meanwhile, back at street level I was holding my ear to the ground when I became aware of a gentle distant rumble, my first ever earthquake may be? Like some early Red Indian scout, I tried to interpret what this could be. The rumble grew ever louder before turning into a roar. At that point I looked up to perceive a truly awesome sight. A whole stampede of bicycles thundering down upon me curb to curb. A tidal wave of two wheeled snorting, puffing, pedalling, flat capped, grey skinned faceless figures relentlessly bearing down on this little defenceless creature. My entire life flashed before me, all two and a half years of it. Oh no! It was the Dick Kerr's factory workers ridin', ridin', ridin' towards my raw hide. Now I know why my mother thought that under the bed was safer.

I closed my eyes and awaited the inevitable crushing of a thousand pneumatic tyres. When suddenly the cavalry arrived and swooped me out of the jaws of death. "John!!!" screamed my mother as in true Superwoman style she scooped me up into her arms and with a whirl of her long pleated skirt she flew me out of danger.

But what of the ghost-riders in the Ellen Street sky, the stampeding bikers? Who or what were they? "Oh I should have remembered" my mother told me. It was the teatime mad dash migration of the Dick Kerr workers rushing home to roost for the night in the Canary Islands just across Garstang road.

Ever since then I never thought much of people who go across the road for their holidays. It was many years later when I could walk and read that I discovered that all the streets over there were named after birds! Some Canaries!

It wasn't long before I was off on my first ever intrepid expedition into the wide world beyond our freshly donkey-stoned front step, down the great Garstang Road, all alone. Mother had used that universal euphemism "John, get from under my feet and go and play out!" So I did! I strolled off down an empty Ellen street, ambled across the busy main road avoiding the tanks and trucks and toddled off down the road leaving behind the Canary Islands and on towards the great edifice of English Martyrs church.

I did not know Mr. Toad by age three, but I must have felt that feeling of the open road ahead and not a care in the world.

I was happily playing this new game of pretend when suddenly this car stopped along side me, its passenger door creaked open and from within its dark cavernous interior a man's voice said "Are you lost little boy? Get in."

Innocently I climbed on to the black ridged running board and hauled my chubby little legs onto the shiny soft dark brown leather seat beside the voice and we shot off at what seemed to me easily as fast as those factory bikers in their impersonation of the Ellen Street 'Ride of the Valkeries'. So, this was a mo- tor- car? Ah, the naivety of childhood!

After what must have seemed a lifetime my mother rang the police from the nearest phone situated in the presbytery of English Martyrs' church declaring a lost child. "Describe him to me" said the stern voice of the police sergeant." "He has blonde curly hair, brown eyes, he is wearing brown sandals, white socks, a white blouse and dark blue short pants", my very worried mother cried.

When she arrived at Preston's main police station she found me sitting happily on top of an ancient, large black enamelled type writer, my little legs dodging the swinging arms of the letters as they spelt out the report of the incident. The agonies we subject our parents to whilst we as children remain oblivious, thinking its all just a magical game.

It was not easy for my mother during those awful war years. My father, Harry, was a fine chap who like thousands of other ordinary but brave men had seen it as their duty to join the armed forces to prevent, amongst other things, us children all becoming little Nazis.

Since my father departed a tearful 172 Ellen Street on a cold winters day in 1939, waved off by my mother, grandfather, grandmother, my sister Pauline and my five aunties and great aunt Annie Burke, my mother had had a tough time. My later attempts to emulate Pooh Bear wandering into the wild woods of Preston was not helping at all, nor was it to improve much either as subsequent escapades showed.

It was a warm sunny day in 1943 whilst visiting my mother's sister, auntie Elsie Jones at her war time prefab in Leyland, that I had been given a rare treat of an ice cream cornet. This was "simply heaven Piglet" as I once again forgot all else and with mum chatting to her sister, Pooh wandered off once again on his tod.

So scrumptious was this amazing treat that I became totally unaware of my immediate surroundings and promptly slid down this large bomb crater on the dusty lane which led to Leyland Motors tank factory. The floor of the hole was covered in fine warm sandy soil and I sat on my bottom still licking my precious ice cream. We had both survived yet another attempt by the enemy to spoil my day.

After that encounter with the enemy all future air raid warnings would be taken seriously and therefore we practiced sheltering under the stairs at 172. I remember it well as I got to wear my special child's gas mask which had a turquoise anodised breathing canister in front, a pink face cover and big goggle eye glasses all strapped tightly to your head with broad rubber bands. I thought Wow, first boy into space !

5

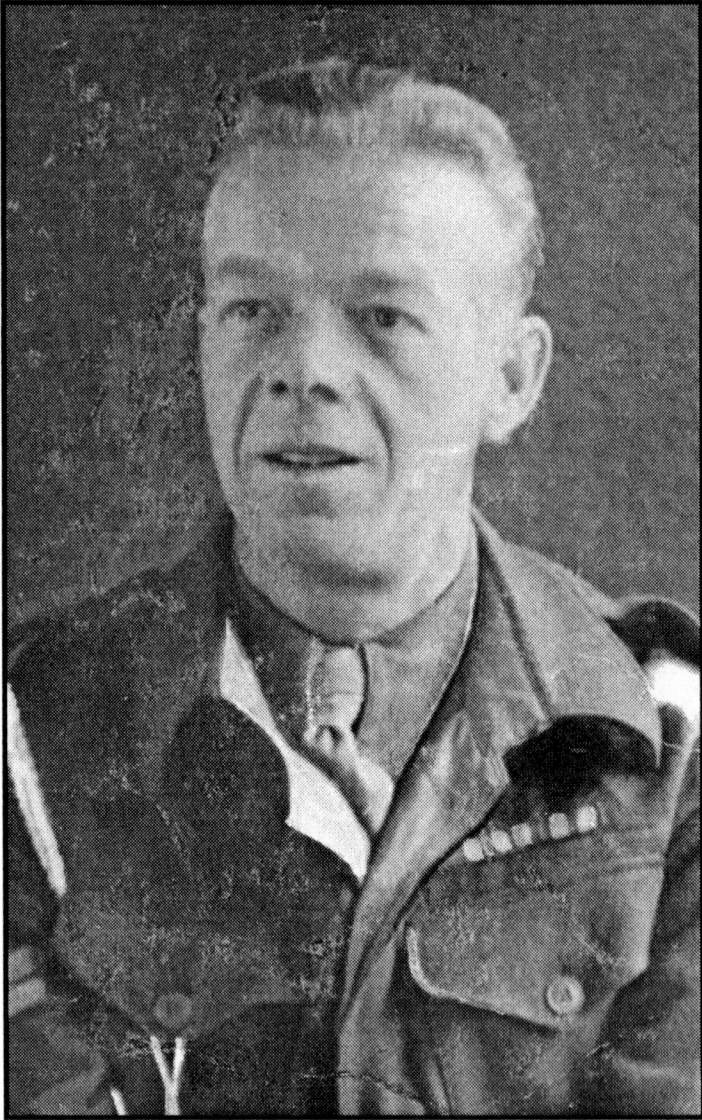

HARRY

Time passed and I grew up believing my mother was my mother and my grandad was my father, although mother constantly told me about my real father, showing me photographs of him somewhere in North Africa or India or Italy or Holland and eventually the Black Forest of Germany. But who was he really?

One morning in 1946 my mother in tears of joy shouted, "Harry is coming home!" I felt an immediate panic of emotions. What would happen to life in Ellen street? What would he be like? What would happen to my cosy world of relationships in my all familiar family forum, my own land of Happy Families? This was a new deal and I was very worried at what had been dealt. Was this my first experience of depression?

This apparition stood motionless before me framed by the shadow of the front door architrave opening onto a bright daylight background which cast his face and figure in momentary mystery. His thin, lined face, sun tanned but sallow, topped by a crop mop of blonde wavy hair contrasted against the tired state of his well worn uniform. Grandad said he had been travelling across war torn Europe for days to reach home. The figure looked very tired. He had survived some of the great battles of the second world war; El Alamein; Sicily; Solerno; Anzio Beach Head; Monte Casino; India; Invasion of Europe; Arnhem; Germany. A new battle of normality was to begin.

The sergeant's stripes blanched against the fading fabric of the khaki battle dress tunic, his steel helmet hung from his left shoulder like a small medieval shield and his ·303 Lee Enfield rifle was slung menacingly across his back. One war worn hand rested on the trigger guard, the other guarded a bulging kit bag containing 'what I wondered!' The home coming had begun.

For a moment this visage of a war weary, battle worn warrior stood motionless on the threshold of 172 Ellen Street, an awesome sight of a complete stranger to this five year old as his son was led slowly towards him clutching tightly his mother's soft warm reassuring hand.

"John" she gently announced, barely concealing her anxiety, "this is your father". We all stood immobile, frozen in one of those eternal time-warped moments when one gets a kind of surreal suspension of what normally passes for life, a microcosm of another existence which runs like some parallel universe unnoticed in the dream which normally passes for life.

It was all too much and I retreated to hide behind my mother's skirts, much to every ones disappointment.

The celebrations lasted well into the night and the entire family of grand parents, aunts and uncles, cousins and friends and Mrs. Penswick, partied like only the Farrons could party. I was plonked on top of the upright piano as Aunty Annie Burke dressed in her standard uniform of long black dress and small floral print pinny, vamped her way through all the old time musicals, all in the same key! The Woodbine fag drooping from her purple lips, its ash defying gravity, added to the theatre of the joyous occasion and not once did she spill a drop of her glass of Guinness, much to the approval of Mary Ellen who would cry, "play it again Annie"!

Then the moment I had been waiting for. The bulging kit bag was opened and out came my present, a magnificent sleek model clockwork metal speed boat brightly painted in silver, with red go faster stripes. I was stunned. Cautiously, my eyes first seeking my mother's approval, I accepted the stunning gift from the soldier stranger as his tired brown eyes sought acceptance in his son's expressionless face.

2 DEPRESSING DARWEN

Life in Ellen Street finally came to an abrupt end with my father's decision to leave his comfortable job as manager of the local CWS store, otherwise known as the Co-op, and buy a medium sized grocery and off-licence shop in the east Lancashire mill town of Darwen.

What a culture shock this was to be!

We moved late in 1946 and in the next year came the terrible winter of 47 when everything froze inside and out. To a six year old this was an amazing experience, especially when my father and I yanked open the frozen tight shop door and I was buried in snow which had drifted high against it. No school today, whoopee!

No, no dreaded St. Joseph's elementary, in-more-ways-than-one, RC school. An ugly Dickensian period Victorian stone monument to all that should have been left there. It was buried deep in a shallow valley and wedged between a formidable high stone escape-proof wall and a narrow back ginnel, along which a refuse littered, industrial swirling foam stream slugged along. My apologies, it might have been the river Darwen!!

It wasn't just the place; it was the foreign language that the poorly dressed, clogged, other children spoke. My sister and I were taunted endlessly about our 'posh' accent. Imagine that, coming from Preston!

The infant and junior schools were administered by Jesuit priests and taught by an order of nuns called Sisters of Mercy – except that they showed none!

Their black Darth Vader style habits enhanced their reign of terror as they glided Dalik like across the bare wooden worn floors to strike with deadly accuracy the back of your little talking head with their solid gold wedding ring. Oh yes, they were married, to Jesus, and by Jesus when that knuckle-duster struck you knew it!

The only warning of incoming was the rustle of their skirts accompanied by the rattle of their long black ivory rosary beads and crucifix. It was rumoured that each bead represented a hit and not a Hail Mary as we were taught in the catechism lesson.

The senior school rated no better with its cruel regimes of discipline enforced by constant fear of arbitrarily administered corporal punishment, and lorded over by a heartless headmaster we called 'Owd Gus' who taught mental arithmetic with the cane. It was no wonder that a slow learner like me developed a lasting block against any form of numbers. I was always in awe of my father who could reckon up a customer's long shopping bill entirely in his head in seconds and wished I could do the same. But I guess my attempts to escape in any way mentally or physically were not really the answer. If only I wasn't so sensitive, such a feeling, artistic little child, deeply devotional and basically soft, I could have braved it all better.

Perhaps the most inspiring moments at St. Josephs were at morning assembly when the whole school sang 'Jerusalem'. This gave me hope to find something that would lift my soul out of this place, surrounded as it was by dark satanic mills. There were fields, somewhere and these were ancient times.

It wasn't that I lacked adventure or courage as my regular sorties across the beautiful Darwen moors often at dusk and alone would show. No it was more a lack of willingness to accept this world as I found it and just get on, rather than always seeking beauty, justice and kindness in place of this other. I knew these qualities existed, they were out there, I had to find them, they had to be there.

I therefore resolved after much brutal realisation of the truth about things that it would be much more pragmatic to adopt the wisdom and advice given by the Roman Emperor and philosopher Marcus Aurelius in his book Meditations, quote: "Begin each day by telling yourself: today I shall be meeting with interference, ingratitude, insolence, disloyalty, ill-will and selfishness - all of them due to the offenders ignorance of what is good or evil."

Perhaps the world was OK? It was just my selective way of looking at it that was wrong; an error of attitude that was to cost me dearly in years to come.

Meanwhile back home in Bolton Road, in order to ensure we did not deliberately oversleep in an attempt to avoid this awful school, my father had hired a truly Dickensian early warning system - the Knocker-Up. This wizened character would rat-tat-tat on your bedroom window for a shilling a week. Alarm clocks had been invented but you could not turn this damned thing off until you switched the bed room big light on and you showed your pale face at the window. And then behold! you saw this Lowry like scene of groups of women, their heads covered in dark shawls clasped around their face, shrouded in the evaporating clouds of their panting breath as it rose into the cold early morning air. The sound of their clogs cantering them down th'hill, t'mill in rhythm with the flickering of their shadows cast by the incandescent pale green glow of the gas light at the corner of the street.

I slept in the store room over the shop. This doubled as my bed room and a loading bay, it housed a giant mechanical crane which loomed large in the corner of the room and in my very active child's imagination. The crane would be used to lift sacks of flour and other goods from adjoining Maria Street into the room by day, but by night it became a Tyrannosaurus Rex, its large jib casting a great shadow with the aid of my bedside Sacred Heart devotional night light candle. Invariably I hid under the bed clothes and created my own little world free from this creeping dark and depressing outside world called Darwen. How I hated this place.

Maria street was not an Ellen street, more of an early Coronation street without the colourful characters, but with all the back-to-back terraced houses with their regimented row upon row of regulation smoking chimneys, cobbled streets, flagged pavements and the obligatory gas lamp. It was however, home to Mrs Smith and her daughter Hilda Smith. They lived in one of the two adjacent tithed terraced cottages on the corner of Maria Street and Bolton Road rented from my father as part of the package he had bought with the business.

Widow Mrs. Smith and her shy spinster daughter were quiet gentle folk who had, like so many northern families fallen on hard times with the loss of their breadwinner and now eked out an existence in the cold cruel climate of austere post war Britain. We liked the Smiths and my father who by nature was a kind and generous man did all he could to help them survive the cruel economic conditions of rationing, austerity and industrial depression.

Hilda was invited to take on the role of nanny to my sister Pauline and me and amongst other things used to take us for walks in Whitehall Park, one of those fine altruistic public works programmes used to employ many out of work men folk during the great depression of the thirties. Then, suddenly, like many strange spontaneous moments in one's life, I remember vividly the rapid onset of this overwhelming mental depression as we passed under the ornate iron Victorian arcade just before we reached the park. I was still only six, where did this come from? Why me? Why now? What was this strange phenomenon? What on earth was this terrible feeling of despair?

As suddenly as it came, it went leaving a sinister marker for future reference.

On Friday evenings, I was allowed to raid the large bottles of sweets in my father's shop without surrendering my sweet rationed points, and go to visit Hilda and her mum in their little terraced cottage. The living room come kitchen was complete with a black polished fire cooking range with one of those fascinating iron bridges on which the large black sooted kettle sat, its steam gently rattling its lid. A stone slab sink with one cold water tap dripped from its perch in the wall and a single gas cooking ring sat on fresh clean newspaper *specially changed in my honour* completed the domestic scene. And all this lit by a single gas light which hissed menacingly through its broken meshed mantle above a cluttered large table covered by a heavy brocaded cloth.

But first the tin bath in front of a blazing coal fire with carbolic soap and scrubbing brush. After all this was Friday night and once a week was not too bad for a boy to suffer, and anyhow what simple fun this really was.

Once dressed the real game was on - the cards were on the table!

Out came the tin box containing the 'money', old buttons of every hue to be our gambling tokens as poker faced we got down to a serious game of Newmarket and other popular card games of the period . No Happy Families here only hard betting to win bags of barley sugars and lemon drops. Hilda and her mum were real professionals, winning most hands with sharp moves, slick fast shuffles and lightning deals. Mrs. Smith, I fancied, wore one of those green croupier's eye shades to evade the gas light distracting her gaze. She certainly seemed to hold all the aces, even the ones I had.

Apart from these, there were other happy days and happy folk in Darwen; it's just that I don't remember them. I seemed to spend all my weekends avoiding reality and escaping back on the bus to Preston, and our relations in the surrounding districts which always seemed warmer, brighter and more cultured. What a snob I was becoming. What a mental escape artist I became and how depressing was the return to Darwen.

And so I resolved to find the Truth, sank all my faith in the Church and became the most impossible, devoutly religious, precocious boy you could meet, much more self righteous than thou or any of you reading this.

And so - Sundays programme would run as follows: 0730 Holy Communion after overnight fast; faint and be carried out by Church Wardens on a regular basis; recover after breakfast; walk back to church to attend 1100 Tridentate Mass and sing solo boy soprano part in Latin whilst trying not to faint again and fall over Choir balcony. Lunch 1pm. Back to church for Baptisms at 2pm [if lucky got paid to sing]; 3pm wander moors till 6pm Benediction back at church; 6.45 go home shouting the odd religious taunt in the door way of the Salvation Army's Redemption Hall as my fellow choir boys and I legged past it. 9 pm to bed with resident dinosaur and my dreams of Utopia and Jerusalem.

Then along came the great threat to my dream world. The 'Eleven Plus' exam. In a perverse sort of way I had always attempted to avoid extra school work by aiming for about sixth place in class course work and therefore not really scholarship grade. On the day of the exam I sat staring out of the windows of Darwen Grammar School at the snow covered hills and dreamt only of how fast I could sledge down them. What a waste of an opportunity, and one that I was to greatly regret when I had to work a forty eight hour week plus four nights a week of night school to gain the necessary qualifications I needed so much for my chosen career. (In later life I would be able to claim I went to Grammar School, just for a day!!) So much for dreams and escapisms. You reap what you sow!

But it was some time before I would really learn this lesson, and in the meantime I would continue with my indulgence in reading tragic heroes and watching black and white melancholic films which sapped my little free consciousness and weakened my already poor character. What a wishy washy wimp, swimming in a sea of despondency I was becoming. I would need to change this soon or drown in it! These kind of mental swamps are the very breeding grounds for the deadly virus 'desponditis'.

Life was not all so bad and indeed most of the holidays were very happy times. Some time with my parents and some time with my relatives who in the main were professional people and in many ways were my source of a private secondary education. I was after all an intelligent, cultured being at my core.

So I learnt English from Aunt Jane who was a school teacher and always asked plumbers how many O levels they had before they were allowed in the house. Fortunately she would correct my bad grammar. She was married to Uncle Walter who was a Factory Manager who used to question me on the entire ingredients of the HP sauce bottle before I was allowed to use it at meal times. Uncle Walter had a brand new Ford Anglia car with shiny new tyres which, when I was younger, would sniff from under the car whilst it was parked outside my Grandmother's house in the now legendary Ellen Street. There where no drugs in those days. To have a car at all during wartime was rare and I used to believe they were incredibly rich. Needless to say, Uncle Walter taught me about the rewards of capitalism and cotton mills including the dark and satanic.

I learned music and Social History from Aunt Elsie who was a fervent socialist and made me read the entire works of Dickens, whilst good old Uncle George, who was an MD of a brewing company, and right of Genghis Khan, would occasionally let me have the odd half pint of his beer. These two were real characters and you could always tell when they had fallen out because Aunt Elsie would storm off into the front room of their 'posh' semi by the river and hammer out the piano solo from Grieg's Piano concerto, puffing furiously on her Capstan Full Strength cigarette whilst in full high dudgeon, calling down unrepeatable curses upon her husband's head. Boy what high passion, what shear raw emotion, what expression of female fire power! 'The Queen of the night versus Zarastro'. All bets were now off.

Drama came from Aunt Anne who managed a high class shoe shop called Lotus & Delta and was highly theatrical, being as the whole family were, thespians and belonged to the Preston Amateur Dramatic Society. I was tutored in Politics by her bespoke suited spouse, Yorkshire man Uncle Jim who was a forty-a-day un-tipped, cigarette chain smoking, senior Civil Servant and as red as the Soviet flag. They had no children of their own so they used to borrow me at holiday times to mow their lawn whilst learning all the parts from Gilbert and Sullivan's operas around their grand piano. I found Marx extremely intellectual but unfortunately completely misleading to the working classes who misinterpreted him in their excuse to be revolting. So much for Socialism!

Enough! Just give me the Good Life. Meanwhile, down on the farm I was to learn all about the Good Life. My Aunt Marie and Uncle Jack were, by complete contrast, down to the real earth and the salt of it to. Holidays on their farm were just magic. This was the life then. Mucking out, shooting rats, feeding pigs, collecting eggs, fishing in pits, milking cows, chasing girls. This intellectual stuff is ok to a point you know, but you can over do it to the point of depression.

Ironically, the depression did not return until some years later after the family had left Darwen and returned to Preston and I had started my apprenticeship in aeronautical engineering at guess where? Yep! English Electric's Dick Kerr works now building jet fighters and bombers.

Now, where are those cyclists?

3 THE APPRENTICESHIP

My introduction to the new world of work was both exciting and bloody. At 0730 hours precisely I rendezvoused with the brass plate screwed to the wall outside the exclusive doorway to the Personnel Department which proudly and officially announced to the world, in splendid copper-plate engraving, that this was the site of the English Electric Company Limited. I had arrived in the awesome world of aeronautics. No more model balsa built bombers for me, this was the real thing.

"Well lad, don't just stand there gawping, come in here", an official voice barked in my ear. In some slow motion like dream state I crossed the brass polished threshold of one of the most famous names in aviation history and on to the parquet wooden corridor floor leading to the Personnel Department waiting room.

"Wait in there laddie", said Reg, the official gate keeper to this exclusive portal from his high stool perch just inside the doorway. Reg was a time served waxworks model works policeman who had earned this prestigious perch of a post and was very proud of it. "Make the most of this moment lad. In future it will be the workers entrance gate for apprentices like you."

And so my private rebellion with officialdom was born and I resolved that one day I would cross both Reg, his petty perch of power and this exclusive threshold on my own terms!

"This is Mr Thompson, he will process your details", said Reg before once more regaining his perch of power. Mr Thompson sat at a simple wooden desk, a thin, pale faced clerk wearing an ill-fitting demob suit with a large illfitting shirt and shiny tie. His black 'short-back-and-sides' hair slicked down with brylcream and parted in the centre. The leather elbow patches on his jacket completed the austere attire and his tired eyes expressed his weary work ethic.

There were four of us starting that April morning and I was allocated my clock number of 63/244. The digits would remain part of my identification throughout my long career with this great company. We were led out of the highly polished parquet floored passage and emerged into a dark tunnel which led to a pair of large rubber flapped doors beyond which the sound of Dick Kerrs hit you as you morphed into the cacophony of riveting guns, windy drills and hammered metal which met our deafened, unaccustomed ears.

Then the sight I had been waiting for, a row of Canberra bomber front fuselages stretching away into the distance, their perspex nose cones reflecting the lights of a hundred pale blue/green argon-arc roof lights. Each pitot head protruding like a short lance draped with its own warning bright red flight safety pennant ready for the charge. Running parallel to the line of Canberra bombers on the opposite side of the passageway was a long continuous sheet-steel barrier impervious to the eye and painted in standard English Electric green. In the centre of this steel screen was a small single opening guarded by a works policeman. I noted that everyone who went in had to show a special yellow security pass for the scrutiny of the guardian of the gate. This mysterious feature immediately caught my eye, so I asked my escort what lay behind this mysterious barrier. "That's the Iron Curtain lad and everything behind it is absolutely top secret". One day, I noted mentally, I would have to penetrate its portals and discover for myself the hidden secrets it contained. I had always fancied myself in the espionage game and a master of disguise dressed in the regulation brown smock which I observed all those who were allowed behind the curtain wore! I would pretend to be the boffin Q!

My daydream was suddenly interrupted by a loud voice "You're here Jones," said our Personnel person, personal tour guide. Oh no! I wanted to start here. I knew about planes, I could name all the parts and one day I would pilot them. But my silent protests went unheard and the remaining apprentices were led away down the long broad central passageway and under the huge banner proclaiming in big letters 'No Spitting'.

We dropped the other two off enroute and after some distance the escort and I arrived at '52 shop' – better known locally as the mad house! We approached a battery of stand drills operated by a group of turbaned wearing women who smiled in formation and silently and critically gave the lad the once over. "You're here" said the escort, then turned and unceremoniesly left the scene.

"Right young man" said the fat man in a light brown smock uniform sitting on a low stool next to an ugly looking giant stapler like machine. "This is a Nibbler and I want you to use it like this, so don your overalls and let's get nibbling", said the Charge Hand.

Overalls? I wasn't prepared for this! My dad had told me to dress smartly and so I was dressed in blue blazer, white shirt, tie and grey flannels. Hardly your blue collar worker's outfit! "Never mind, sit here and push these DFTs up against these cutting jaws like this", he said. A Drilling and Filing Template (DFT) was a hardened balfour steel sandwich with layers of razor sharp duraluminum cropped sheets as the filling. The Nibbler then knawed away as you applied pressure against the teeth chattering machine.

A lifetime later I arrived home, my smart outfit covered in fine oily smelling compo and aluminium dust, my hands bleeding from a thousand tiny cuts and my ears ringing with the nightmare noise of the Nibbler.

However, properly dressed, I got used to my temporary stay in the 'mad house' although some of the practices were very risky by todays safety standards and reinforced the notion of the time that apprentices were expendable!

Such was the attitude then, you would be sent to the chemical treatment shop nearby to carry out a variety of simple but potentially deadly tasks like degreasing metal components in a deep tank of trichloroethylene. Being a short lad I had to lean precipitously over the side of the tank to lower my wire mesh basket of items tied to a rope down through the rising fumes of the boiling mixture. As you did so you could not help breathing in some of the stray mist that came up to meet you. The effect was like an instant high from anaesthetic gas, you became light headed, and now balancing on tip toes teetered on the brink of falling in and that would have certainly taken the shine out of your Brylcreamed hair do.

On another occasion I was told to climb up into the open jaws of a large hydraulic press which had an upper male and a lower female steel moulding tool bolted to each bed. Equipped with a bucket of whale oil I was instructed to grease the two mating surfaces from within side the press! It was nasty and awkward work and the oil stunk.

Since one had to lie on your back to complete the job it could have entirely reshaped your career had the on button been accidentally pressed.

The whole world of work was punctuated by endless characters. Some I liked, some I loathed. Some I detested for their total lack of culture. Some where so banal I wrote poems about them.

Men like machines or like automatons,
Breathed without air,
Lived without mind, thought without head,
No soul had they to bare.
This was the land of the living,
But these were the mentally dead.

But somehow you survived and as long as you kept your sense of humour there were some good fun times and you did learn a lot about people, life and, oh yes, aeronautical engineering.

On one occasion whilst working on the Top Secret TSR2 (successor of the Canberra TSR1) I was to find a start to my parallel career. At age fifteen I joined the Air Training Corps and by sixteen I was a solo pilot. This was to be the beginning of a lifetime of aviation, civil and military, which I have now enjoyed for fifty years.

Aviation was to be my life and to provide me with a cadre of friends, lifestyle, a good living and some of the happiest days and greatest adventures in it. It was also to teach me a great deal about my self and the secret of being in the present moment and what vitality the rediscovery of that which had been forgotten in childhood. The sheer, exhilarating, venture adventure, the beginning of another Biggles, yes! After being catapulted to a thousand feet over the white cliffs of Dover in an open cockpit Kirby Cadet glider with nothing but a bit of ply wood between me and the English Channel, I realised just what I had let myself in for!

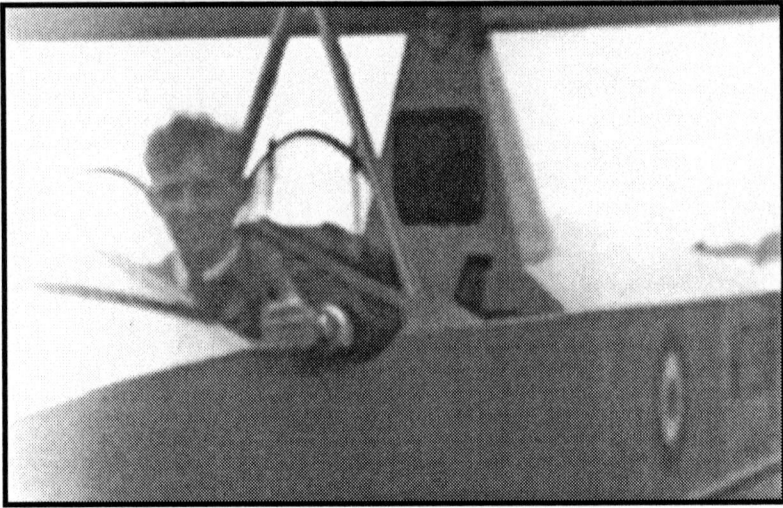

SOLO AT SIXTEEN

My father who had fought at the battle of Arnhem in Holland had seen dozens of troop carrying gliders crash with many fatalities and therefore any mention of gliders would obviously have been met with a definite "No Go". So I had lied to my father, telling him a half truth, that it was in fact a summer camp which I was attending somewhere in England.

If you have ever read the story of Jonathon Livingston Seagull you will know what I mean about the magic of flying and the discovery of ones self, especially the passage in which the wise old bird, Chiang, uses the dynamics of flight to teach his pupil about life, selflessness, and inner wisdom.

I wanted to be like Jonathon. I wanted to learn what he was learning from Chiang.

Meanwhile, my own learning about life and its meaning continued as part of my apprenticeship. That is until around my eighteenth year when 'IT' returned. This time it also was much stronger and lasted for a month or two. This time also it became a very real steady feeling of depression and made everything difficult to handle, especially work, home and social life. What is this awful thing? Why does it come? What's the reason? I never did find answers. I just suffered it. Perhaps it was because I used to ponder a lot on the meaning of things – who am I really? What is this Creation? What is my purpose in it? What's it all about?

These questions would haunt me until I turned twenty one and had graduated to the Drawing and Planning Office. Now this gave me something to really think about! The larger questions persisted though, and I pursued my quest to find answers to the great innate questions of life.

4 SHIRLEY

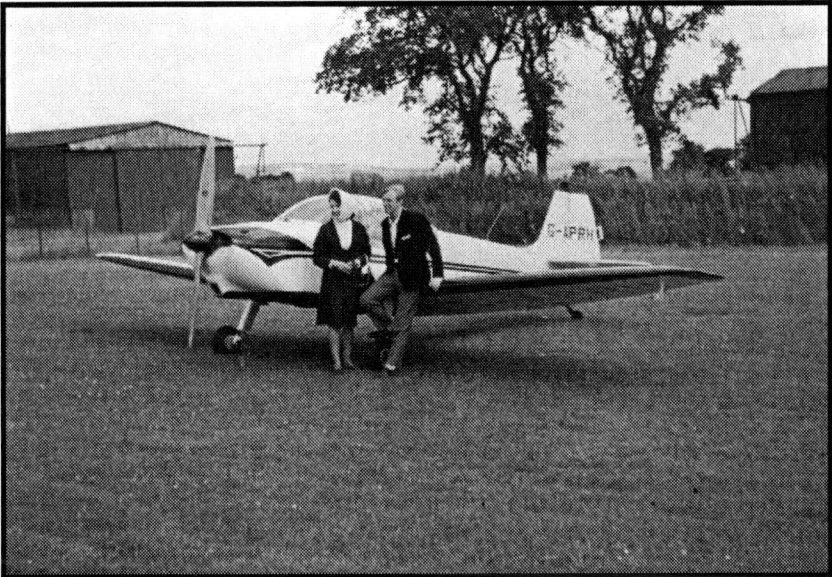

HAPPY HOLIDAYS WITH SHIRLEY AND 'ROMEO HOTEL'

Meeting Shirley had quite an impact on the course of my life and the developing partnership had a profound effect upon my psyche. Instead of flying solo, I had at last found someone who could help me navigate the vicissitudes of life and weather the storms it inevitably brings.

So naturally I taught her to fly, bought a share in a lovely two-seater light touring aircraft with the magic name of 'Garland Bianchi Fairchild Linnet'- the names recording its pedigree; Italian, American and English! What fun we had on our aerial odyssey around the UK and the continent. What a romance. Even the aircraft's phonetic call-sign was 'Romeo Hotel'. Our adventures would at least fill another few chapters, if not another book.

Well another chapter was about to unfold. Shirley and I had been married for seven very happy years. We had two lovely boys, Richard aged five and Andrew aged three when, shortly before our daughter Elizabeth was born, I became ill with an especially virulent form of flu which completely grounded me. Each day the condition worsened as I became gripped in a fever which pushed me into periods of delirium.

Shirley was by now almost full term in her pregnancy and the burden of nursing me was beginning to tell as the fever always seemed to be worse at night. Hospital was considered but there was an epidemic of the illness nationally and so we thought we would try to weather the storm by taking the prescribed medicine at home.

I had moved into the front spare bedroom a week before the birth with all the symptoms of full influenza gradually developing a raging fever as the condition worsened and my grip on consciousness slowly slipped until one night I just wanted to let go. I faintly remember the moment as in the dim bedside light Shirley bent over me comforting me and placing cold towels on my forehead. There was poignancy about that moment in which one was suspended in a sort of ante room between life and death lit by an ethereal light and free of all fear. Everything seemed to be so peaceful and painless and nothing seemed to matter anymore.

I was on the threshold of another place populated by stillness and warmth, a sort of suspended animation of nothing yet everything, division less, all encompassing, still beyond all forms of human imagination, full of bliss and happiness.

Sometime later I must have passed into sleep only to be awoken by the cries of a baby coming from the other bed room. In my semiconscious state I tried to re-enter the world of before and re adjust all my senses to it before succumbing once again to the sleep of this world. Where I had been I know not, but I did know that things from now on things would somehow never be the same again.

The next day I was informed by my mother and mother-in-law that we had been blessed by the birth of a daughter and that if I should continue to improve I would be allowed to see her soon. So after a couple of days I was allowed in my pyjamas and dressing gown to see my wife and my daughter in the next room in what seemed a sort of dreaming state of unreality. Had this really happened whilst I had been to this other place? Or was that the reality and this the dream?

All this ethereal stuff was nicely replaced by the gentle but down to earth reality of our best friends visit and the bed room party which followed. Robert and Margaret had called to welcome the new arrival and great joy and much laughter was enjoyed that day.

That night Shirley began to feel very unwell and in the timeless zone I seemed to inhabit at the time I could hear raised voices in a heated exchange. The doctor had been called and was telling her that there was nothing the matter with her, that it was just the after effects of giving birth and nothing needed to be done. I had a very bad feeling about this and later that day, still dressed in my pyjamas and dressing gown, I felt well enough to sit up with my wife in her bed room to try to comfort her.

Shirley sat very quietly by the bed room window sewing. She seemed strangely remote and only spoke to acknowledge my presence. She was dressed in a long black dress and her mood seemed resigned and subdued in stark contrast to the joy of the recent celebration of the birth of our daughter. She clearly did not accept the doctor's arbitrary diagnosis. Very concerned, not knowing what to do, I returned to my sick bed and eventually went to sleep with a heavy heart.

The next day I awoke late and was suddenly jerked into motion by Shirley's cries for help. She was in bed cradling the baby in her arms and clearly struggling to breathe. I placed our daughter into the cot and desperately tried to comfort my wife in her distress. My mother called 999 and they rushed us both into hospital, Shirley in one ambulance, me in a wheel chair, in another directly behind.

A few hours later Shirley was dead.

Some eternity later, after the effects of the tranquilizers and the anti-biotics had worn off and the last effects of the virus I had suffered and from which my wife had died, faded, there came a new order of trial; the care of the children; Richard 5, Andrew 3 and Elizabeth 2 weeks old. My family were just so good but it was during the early hours of the morning that the darkest thoughts drifted silently and most stealthily into my mind.

One night both boys had been very sick and I had to completely change their beds and resettle them with soothing stories. Having returned to my room, the baby who was lying in the Moses basket at the foot of my bed, awoke for her four am feed.

It was just beginning to come light with that beautiful quality of serenity that comes with an early spring dawn and as I cradled her in my arms we felt the gentle presence of her mother in the room. It was an utterly still and poignant moment of complete stillness. Just then, Andrew and Richard crept quietly in to join us, climbed on to the bed next to me and asked "where is mummy, daddy?" My heart, already broken with their mother's death, was now over whelmed as I lost the struggle to maintain my composure. The pale light in the room, gently grew brighter, and by now exhausted and huddled together, we succumbed to deep sleep.

Sleep on now John for soon the dark night of depression will surely return and with it another chapter, another story of what follows the tragic part of this tale.

Well, that's another story. A story of how you can cope with bringing up a young family as a single father if you have a great family of friends and relatives as I did. Remarkable people like Iain and Angela who took us into their home and helped me to look after the boys like they were their own, whilst I fought off the endless heart break and depression. Wonderful people like my sister Pauline and her husband Peter, Robert and Margaret McNeill who became second parents to baby Elizabeth whilst I returned to work. During this time Richard, my eldest son, grew in manly stature to help me run the family affairs in his own way, always seeking to take on more responsibilities than was really his time to shoulder. Who knows why these things are meant to be, but one question you can always ask is "What can we learn from this? Richard certainly found a steep learning curve up which he climbed with determination and great credit.

These were interesting times and a lot of credit is rightly due to all those extraordinary people who provided unstinting support through out a period of what was undoubtedly a melting pot for the alloys of mind and emotions. These were to lay the future foundation of one's ability to survive the slings and arrows of outrageous fortune with the knowledge that every thing happens for a reason, and so the best attitude to adopt is to ask the question, what is to be learnt from this?

5 ANDREW'S ACCIDENT

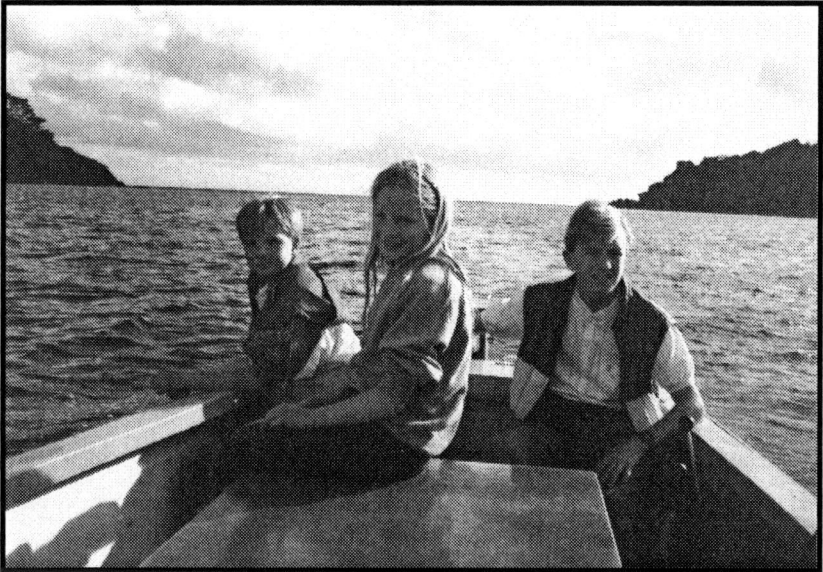

RICHARD, ANDREW & ELIZABETH

CORNWALL HOLIDAY ONE WEEK BEFORE ANDREW'S ACCIDENT

I kissed my mother goodbye and gave my final instructions to the boys about their behaviour and fulfilling their duty to attend their respective Cadet Corps activities on the next day, before setting off for RAF Syerston and my Gliding Instructor's course.

Monday, 9th September dawned bright and heavy dew had settled on the grass lawns surrounding the Officer's Mess as I strolled across to breakfast from the annexed accommodation with my fellow instructor Peter Leggett. We joked about the first day of the course. How, in flying times, an hour under pressure in the air can seem like three on the ground; "It could be a long day", I laughed.

Monday the 9th was for me to be the longest day. By dawn the next day, nothing in this life would ever be the same! Once again my comfortable dream would be abruptly broken by the ever changing face of fate.

The one thing about flying is that it demands your full attention and you are soon reminded of that if you are no longer in the present or in control. Like all potentially hazardous activities, flying an aircraft means constant awareness of what is going on now, and day dreaming, inner conversations and indulgencies into the normal mental fog of 'thinking about things' is not only a waste of time but positively dangerous.

As a young boy I had often found myself avoiding distress by escaping from reality, or situations in which I did not wish to take part by these seemingly harmless mental processes of escapism. Up there a momentary drift into unawareness could cost you your life. I liked the discipline and certainty it brought. No shades of dreamy grey – just black and white. Get it right or you know you have got it wrong instantly.

The first day's flying training to become an instructor was complete and, feeling pleased with my progress, I joined my colleagues in the bar for the traditional unofficial debrief, allowing the alcohol to take its effect on the facial muscles that the nervous laughter had not yet dispelled.

There followed the usual slightly exaggerated stories about how each pilot had handled the difficult moments, how relying on self confidence, each had remained cool, detached, in control – that sort of thing. I allowed myself a moment to dream, after all it was not far to fall from a bar stool! Confident of myself, in control, present, enjoying the reality. This was better than any dream. This was great. This was life. Then I remembered the others and rejoined their presence around me.

Funny, how you drift off from the present whenever ego plays.

"Who's for another? Nowhere to drive tonight John" In an uncharacteristic display of self discipline, I declined. "Got to study for the ground exams and brush up my meteorology, principles of flight and instructional patter" I said, in such a plausible way that my colleagues let me go without a single protest. Most uncharacteristic for aircrew!

It was about 8pm as I strolled back to my quarters in the annexe. The warm September sun painting the trees and lawns with a beautiful ochre and pink. Everything looked good and I enjoyed the evening air and that wondrous stillness that is universally present at dawn and sunset.

I had been studying steadily for about an hour and a half when there was a tap on the window. It was Peter, "There is a message for you at Reception. They said it was urgent." And he disappeared. When I reached the mess I found the bar empty except for the barman who handed me a scribbled note which simply read 'Squadron Leader Farron – Andrew - accident - Richard.'

Unable to contact Richard, I quickly threw a few things in a bag, then, with extraordinary calmness rang friends at home to check if any hospital had admitted Andrew. He was finally tracked down to Blackburn Royal Infirmary with multiple fractures and severe head injury. His chances of survival were apparently very poor. There was a possibility of his transfer to Salford hospital for a brain scan but his condition was considered too unstable for the move. The advice was for me to set off on the 150 mile journey and to call them every half hour for an update.

The journey home was quite extra ordinary if not surreal and was guided by a power as though from above.

For the next fifteen years what followed is quite an interesting and remarkable tale of extraordinary development and transition of personal character through a highly emotional and exacting trial of the ability to overcome adversity and one's allocated lot in life, or perish in the attempt.

During this time I learnt a lot about everything, about life and death. About people, family and friends. About the medical profession, and the farcical and temporal nature of our ideas of 'my life' and the real value of things. Most of all, I learnt about myself. Who I was, and more important, who I was not. How you can be or not be and the difference between the two. How never to take no for an answer, no matter who should say the negative. How to realise that nothing is impossible, after all I am limitless ! And so I was.

Once resolved to meet the situation and accepting it (fully) the gods come to your aid. Here I was with this broken boy; this crumpled child; this seriously injured son. There it was, the situation and I needed to deal with it. No time for self pity now, no time for me, no time to be other than present.

I will never forget the moment of crystallization, that explosion in consciousness, when I was told by the Hospital doctor that "that was all they could do". "What usually happens to your brain damaged children" I asked? "Oh, they usually die!" What an ignition of power this sparked inside me. What a surge of energy this simple statement of truth caused. "Well, this is one child who will not die and what's more, we will be back to show you" I bellowed in outright defiance against this bland statement of convention.

Andrew remained in a coma for 3 months before the first sign of recovery. During that time I had learnt very quickly about brain damaged children and that there were little or no special paediatric facilities available. With the help of Andrew's Sea Cadet unit (from which he had been cycling home on the night of the

34

accident) I mounted a determined campaign to do everything possible and impossible to save my child.

Lieutenant Commander Gordon Cadman RNR and the Chorley Sea Cadets were fantastic. After Andrew had been moved out of the Intensive Care unit but still in coma, the cadets would travel the thirty miles to the Manchester Children's Hospital every evening to visit him. They dressed in their uniforms in an attempt to spark some response and surrounded his bed gently speaking to him about what they had done together on that night before the fateful accident. Their help was invaluable and we owe a lasting debt of gratitude to them for their help then and in the special treatment which Andrew was to need later.

Three years later, free of his wheelchair, Andrew walked into the same childrens' ward of his own accord. Five years later he was to graduate from college with IT qualifications. Six years later he was to start work. Fifteen years later he was to look after me during the worst depression of my life!

How did this miracle happen?

Well that's another story too; Andrew's story.

It contains amazing tales of what can be achieved by applying mind over matter and learning not to take no for an answer. Of how to research, plan, project manage, fund, publicise the effects of your son's tragic accident and turn it from a disaster to his advantage. Of how to use all the emotions to help your cause for justice and how to plan, strategise, survive and succeed in winning essential compensation for major injuries from the Insurance industry against all the odds and their intransigence. How to survive six years of relentless attrition to win your case, and win it with indefatigable energy, humour, tenacity and a vision. You gotta have vision!

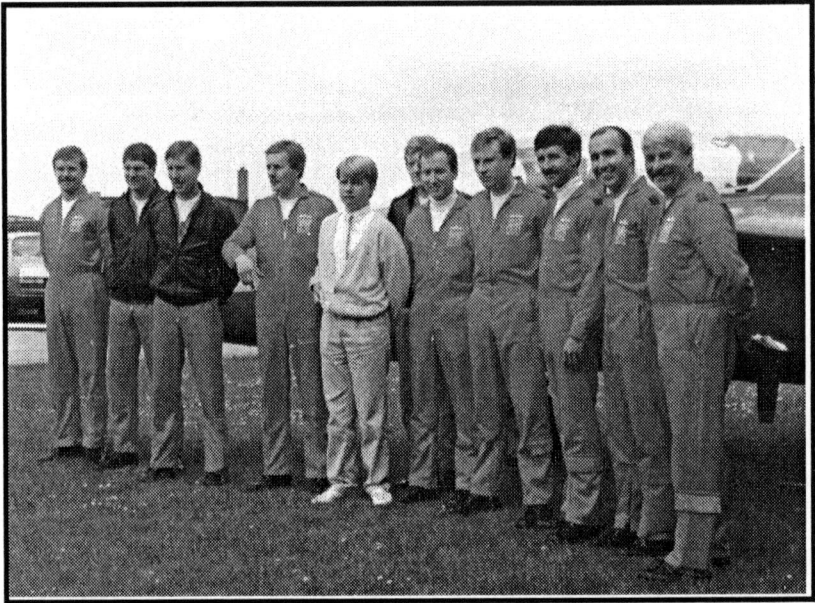

THE RED ARROWS HELP ANDREW'S RECOVERY

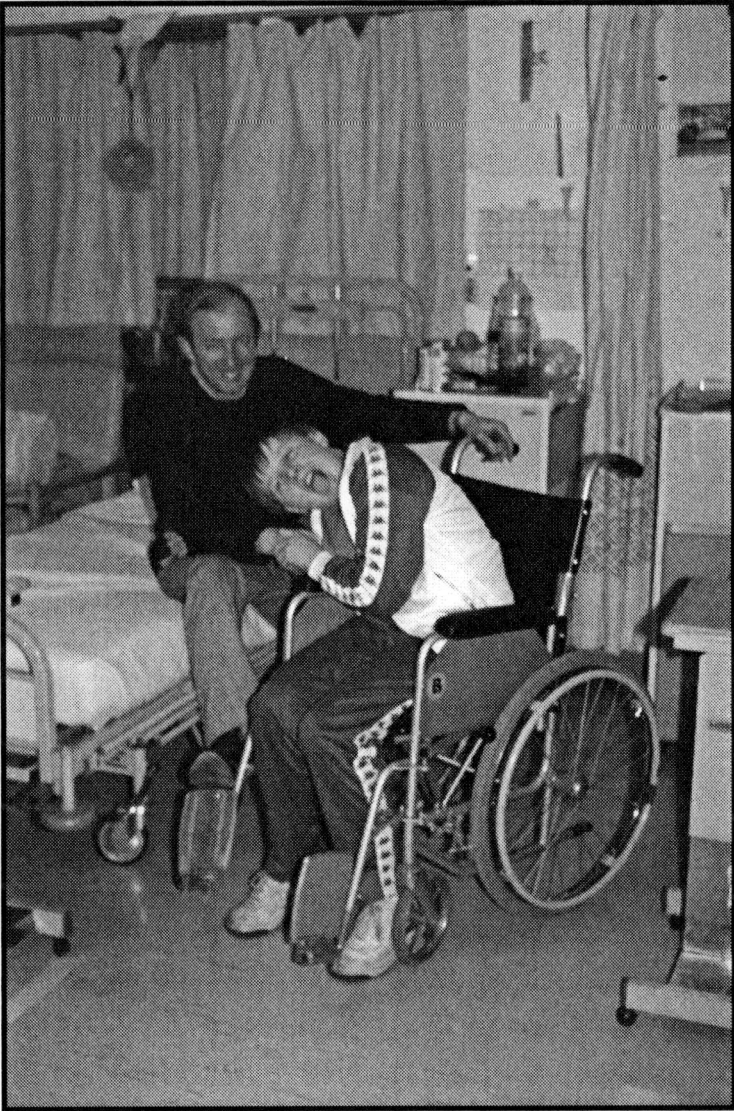

Andrew in recovery phase

6 TIPPING THE BALANCE

FINGER ON THE TRIGGER

Every one will be familiar with the 'Trigger Principle'. You know, there are the right conditions for something to happen. There are the right ingredients, there are the right circumstances, there are the right people and the right confluence of the stars and there is the nature of the individual. All we need now is a trigger and BANG! The fragile truce of our prevailing emotional state is blown asunder.

Well it's just the same with the 'tipping point' of the entry into deep depression. Usually one is unaware of the conditions surrounding this point, although they maybe obvious to others and so, unless the warnings are heeded, it is very likely that the finger is unwittingly on the trigger and all we need is that fatal catalyst from which the trigger, once pulled there is no dragging back the bullet that will strike our own heart with such devastating effect. The balance has tipped.

And so it was in my case, a classic example of just those critical moments - the tipping point or the trigger to set the whole process off. So the scene is set and all the aforementioned conditions are in place, the year 2000.

The beginning of the new millennium was to have been the great opportunity for a number of new and exciting projects such as the proposal to fly three of our aircraft around the United Kingdom, visiting every Squadron. This was named the Millennium Falcon and the project had been officially launched by His Royal Highness Prince Philip at the 1998 Farnborough Air show.

Naturally such a high profile event had attracted a great deal of attention, both from the aerospace industry, the Air Cadet Organisation and the press. Not to mention of course the personal interest His Royal Highness was taking in the project as Commandant in Chief of the Air Training Corps. I was designated as Project Officer and as such had responsibility for ensuring liaison with Buckingham Palace and all the formations involved in the undertaking. Co-incidentally I was also responsible for our cooperation with a major international aerospace group and its input into the Royal International Air Tattoo which was being moved from its original base at RAF Fairford to a new venue at RAF Cottesmore. All this was causing a great deal of pressure in the build up to these events and was steadily creating a very stressful working environment.

Major events of this kind are incredibly exciting, full of challenges and fuelled by high octane adrenaline and whilst terrific in their thrill of uncertainty they are naturally flown at high emotional 'angles of attack'. The risk factor of potential screw up or high visibility failure is constantly causing you to re calibrate your instruments and crucial orientation. Let's see now, are we straight and level or inverted? Climbing or descending, yawing or rolling? Must check my altitude, speed, track . What's my heading? What's the Outside Air Temperature? Oh no! Ice on my wings! Where on earth did I arrange for the Red Arrows aircraft mock up to be situated? When will the Secretary of State for Defence arrive and what will be his questions?

By this time the gyroscopic instruments of your mind that tells you which way is up have toppled. Your inner ear deceives you. Disorientation claims your belief and you are about to enter a spin. Your grip on the control column of life drains the blood from hands and you are on the 'white knuckle ride'. How did all this come about?

In January of that year I had attended my routine annual RAF/CAA flying medical, and when undergoing the ECG test the doctor noted a very small blip on the scan. "Better have this checked with Central Medical Establishment" said the doc and duly referred me to the Cardiology Department at Peterborough General Hospital for an appointment some weeks later. No problem I thought. I have been flying military and civilian aircraft for forty years and never failed a medical yet.

So in April, deciding to combine the appointment with a meeting at nearby RAF Cottismore to discuss the company's participation in the Royal International Air Tattoo, I drove down south with full confidence. En route I became acutely aware of an increasing level of anxiety.

RIAT 2000 as the Tattoo was known, was a big responsibility and on top of Farnborough Air Show these commitments were preying on my mind much more than I realised. The deadly clouds of doubt had begun to form in the convection of the mental heat now being generated by the worry of the 'what if?' scenario. I was almost at the end of the journey when I was suddenly overcome by a massive wave of uncontrollable emotion. I pulled into a nearby lay-by and was immediately engulfed in floods of tears. What on earth was this all about? I asked. Where did this come from??? Grown men just don't act like this, do they? I asked of my self in an embarrassing way. If only I had been able to recognise or others had been able to spot the build up of high emotional stress caused by the pressure of work, we may never have arrived at the tipping point.

But with the amazing ability to achieve 20/20 vision after the event even a pilot's highly developed peripheral vision could not see this 'incoming'. At Cottesmore not everything had gone to plan. There were a lot of unknowns, a lot of uncertainties, lots of loose ends. One could feel the clouds of doubt, deadly doubt creeping in. The storm was gathering.

I arrived at the hospital, registered with the RAF Medical Officer and was sent for a 'treadmill test'. During the preliminary ECG wiring up process they take you through I joked with the nurse who told me she had once worked for the Civil Aviation Authority (CAA). Ah! I quipped. The 'Campaign Against Aviation'. Well no problem here then. Just a "walk in the park, piece of cake" I joked, in that typically cocky way aircrew often use to shore up their self confidence in hostile airspace, and promptly stepped onto the tread mill machine.

As the speed increased I began to experience sharp chest pains which correspondingly registered on the ECG monitor screen like warning signs of high oil pressure just before engine failure. These signs seemed to register with my trained thinking and the cursory way of examining a problem in the air like it was the usual EFATO. You know, engine failure after take off, a routine which all instructors had engraved on the Flight Reference Card of their heart. Alpha 662, Roger that Eagle Base? We have an interesting situation here! Am monitoring data and will advise. Stud 3. Go! Have Crash Rescue Vehicle on stand by.

Determined not to fail the test, I gritted my teeth and told myself it was just me being 'unfit'. More speed followed until I could not take the pain anymore, hit the eject button and virtually collapsed at the feet of the medical staff. "Sorry old boy, you have acute angina." echo, echo, echoed in my ears until I came back into the present after the shock wave settled.

I sat for sometime still in a state of shock and disbelief, the words ringing in my ears like a death knell. 'Death' followed shortly afterwards when the Medical Officer pronounced me 'GROUNDED'.

This loss of my 'flying life' was the tipping point into the deadly, deep dive into the Great Depression.

7 THE GREAT DEPRESSION

(THE GREAT ESCAPE / THE DARKEST HOUR)

The Great Escape

It was 6am on Wednesday the 12th July 2000. A brilliant sunny summer's day had dawned. The West Pennine Moors sparkled with the sharp stroke of the morning sun shining through a cloudless azure sky. The birds sang out the last of the morning chorus and all of nature shone like a precious jewel set in the verdant velvet of the Withnell Forest spread out like a royal robe awaiting the monarch of the earth. This was the view from my study window high in the roof of my terraced cottage in the local village.

My appointment with my Chief of Staff, Group Captain Mike Cross at the HQ Air Cadets Royal Air Force, Cranwell, Lincolnshire, was focussing my preparations and directing my actions. Last minute assembly of the reports on progress with three major events were checked and problem issues highlighted for urgent discussion. There were some worrying developments and I could feel the pressure mounting as the solar heating began to raise the temperature in the study. I was only too well aware that these major national and international events were very prestigious and important. High profile, mission impossible, short timescale, problematic project were my stock in trade and I had a good reputation for sorting, solving and delivering.

The organisation I worked for was very professional, world class and I was very proud to work for the top man and loved the buzz of all that adrenaline when times were tight. But today, I was tired through many nights of lack of sleep and unknown to myself my batteries were running flat and my subtle fuel gauge almost empty. I was dangerously close to the stall and the inevitable spin that, even for this experienced pilot, would inexorably follow.

Lurking behind all this business and surface activity was a low but steady frequency of anxiety and fear of failure which had been constantly suppressed and controlled. That was until now. Now it was beginning to break out with flashes of nervous thought, feelings of nausea and a heavy emotional dampness which attempted to cover all my being with a black dark, suffocating blanket of doubt, deadly doubt.

Doubt? This was impossible; I never doubted my abilities and any such doubts were always cut dead with the sharp sword of reason which had always guarded me from such attacks. Today was different; today I could barely conceal the high tide of blackness wanting to extinguish all hope, all light, all faith in myself.

I looked out of the window again across the sleeping neighbourhood, the houses, the little houses with little people, little worlds, some still sleeping, some stirring, some moving, but all completely oblivious to my plight, my pain, my desperation. Could no one help me? I cried out in the blind deafness of my mind. Help me ! Help me for Gods sake, somebody hear my cries!

No one did, my pain was personal, private, unfelt and unknown to others. How could they? I reasoned. How could they know in their own private pools of personal dreaming state, of occasional moments of fleeting consciousness like pin pricks of light in an otherwise uniform greyness of being. In life we are all in the midst of death Christ once said. How true.

I glanced at the clock on my desk; 0615, time to go John! Time to pick up my pre packed pilots portfolio, specially widened briefcase, bags of bumph. I started down the steep, narrow-winding spiral staircase which screwed downwards, reminiscent of a spin. I was in a spin, rotating ever earthwards, out of mental control drawn down by the weight of my briefcase. The handrail turning downwards seemed ever lower and flimsy relative to my descending c of g and accelerating mass. I looked over the rail to the open space and drop of some 15 feet below me.

I had noticed, previously when performing aerobatics and especially in an aerial spin how time seems to slow right down. The adrenaline pumps and the mind, like some detached observer reads out to you the parameters, the toppled gyroscopic instruments, the altimeter winding itself backwards towards zero in some whizzing anti-clockwise motion. Would I acknowledge the direction of rotation? Would I remember to ignore the inner ear telling me to oppose the direction of the spin with aileron or select opposite rudder? Would I remember to push the control column forward rather than yanking it back as my senses were demanding? Would I remember to stabilize the plunging craft until I had recovered flying speed and eased out of the resulting dive.

Would I allow the weight of my heavy briefcase to simply unbalance the carefully, conscious, control of my descent down the spiral stairs (or would I pull out of the spin)? No one would know. It was an accident. He slipped on the shiny wooden slats on the staircase, they would say. The heavy case obviously pulled him over the edge; he broke his neck in the ensuing fall. His wife and young son still asleep would not be able to save him. What a tragedy! What a waste! What an end! Crashed and burned!

They say that just before death, your whole life passes before you. Yes my life . Was this to be it then? The last of a train of tragic events which had dogged my existence so far. My first young wife dying shortly after the birth of our daughter leaving me with the week old baby and our two sons aged five and three.

Then my youngest (at the time) son, then thirteen, being hit by a car whilst he was cycling home one September evening, receiving multiple breakages and severe head injuries which left him with 80% brain damage, on a life support machine and in a coma. The terrible trauma of an idyllic summer holiday in Portugal (with my second wife, Kathryn, daughter Elizabeth and young son James) that turned into a horror story of medical bungling which almost cost me my life and ended with me being aero medically evacuated back to a UK hospital. Perhaps it was as well that I did not know at the time that there were even more to challenges to come. Like the heart attack, the double/triple heart by-pass and most recently my surviving a horrific mid-air collision.

But just now on this sunny morning in June 2000, I was fighting to regain control of my life as my grip on it was rapidly slipping from me. I began to experience a steady, remorseless sense of panic, an inescapable and suffocating sense of despair creeping inexorably over my entire being; a realisation of complete and utter desolation, despair and a deep and profound sadness and depression. You know, unless you have experienced this personally, you simply cannot know the terrible terror of its effect on your body, mind and soul; your being.

I finally reached my car, loaded up my cases, climbed into the driving seat and immediately slumped at the wheel completely overcome with despair and despondency. How long I was there for I cannot remember but having summoned all my remaining strength I drove out towards my destination. On the way I approached my GP's surgery and in a final gasp of desperation decided to seek help, medical advice, admit something was wrong, give in to the perceived shame that I was suffering a nervous break down and possibly mental illness. Something took control and I swung the car into the empty car park, took a deep breath and dragged myself to the reception demanding with forcefulness to see my doctor at once.

He was aware of my condition since there had been clear warning signs some six months earlier when I had felt the depression coming on, inexorably, insidiously, inescapably being born in my mind like the birth of a deadly cancer which I then knew with great foreboding must come to pass. Although sympathetic, he seemed to me not to really be making the right responses and I initially took his attitude to be more of the "pull your self together mode". Well if I could I would and would not be here desperately seeking help! This view was of course untrue, he was trying to help but this business of deep depression is so difficult to understand, to correctly diagnose and prescribe for.

Seeing my pathetic condition though, he very kindly cancelled all his immediate appointments to give me his full attention. With the aid of a diagram he explained how he understood what the causes could be. These symptoms and causes are shown in the following diagrams:

DIAGRAM OF CAUSES

Causes

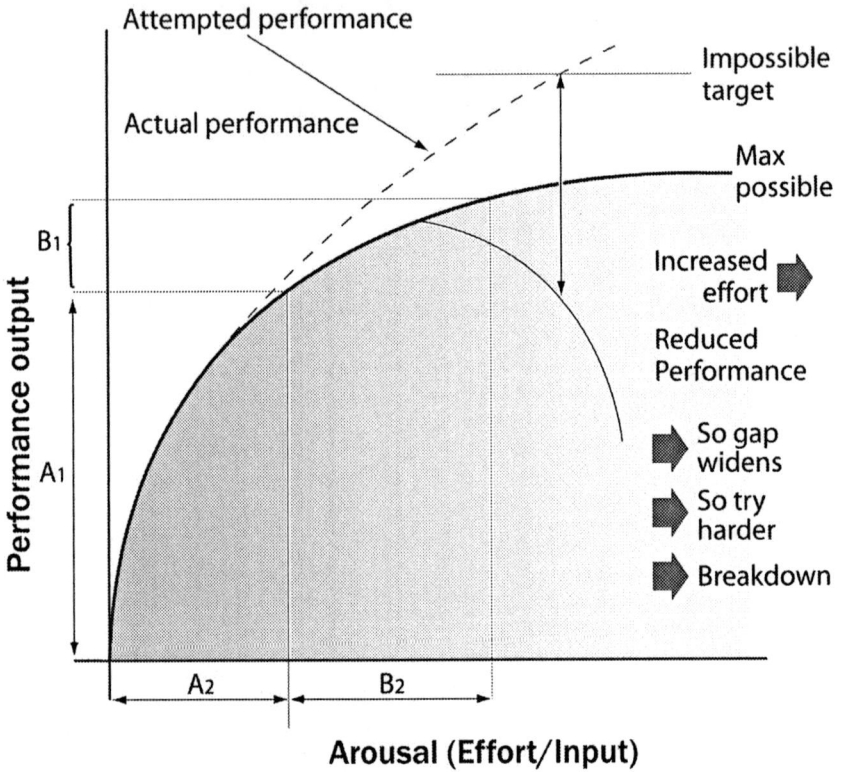

Attempted performance

Actual performance

Impossible target

Max possible

B₁

Increased effort ➡

Reduced Performance

So gap widens ➡

So try harder ➡

Breakdown ➡

Performance output

A₁

A₂   B₂

Arousal (Effort/Input)

$A_{1/2}$ = Efficient - ie 1 unit of effort = 1 unit of performance

$B_{1/2}$ = In efficient contingency reserve -
ie 4 units of effort = 1 unit of performance

$A_{1/2}$ = "Fair days work for a fair days pay" -
with a sensible contingency reserve

Acknowledgements to Dr. Vincent Mainey GP

48

Causes - the Flying Analogy

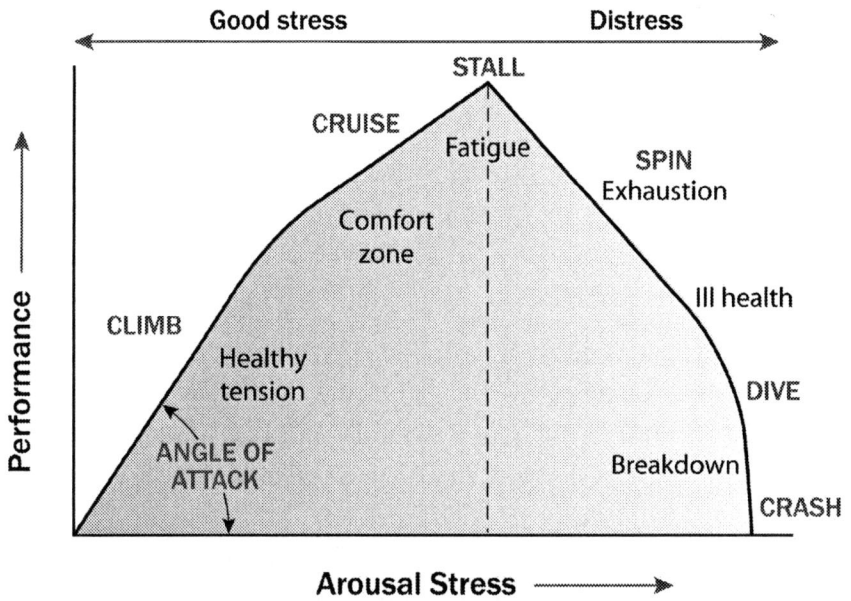

It is all to do with the levels of stress we subject our mind and body to. There is Good stress and there is Distress, and the problem comes at an individual crisis point where the stress peaks and fatigue sets in and mental distress is turned into exhaustion. Ill health and breakdown rapidly follow. So much for the science but what about my immediate and present condition?

We agreed to cancel my business appointments with my Chief of Staff and concentrated on trying to deal with the problem before us. Now an interesting situation arose, the question of my balance of mind became my GP's foremost concern and this led inevitably towards the question of suicide! Had it occurred to me? Had I thought about it? Had I contemplated it? Well in all honesty yes, yes and yes! In that condition every one does. Ask yourself how many times have you felt 'suicidal'?

Bad day, bad cold, bad hair, bad debts, bad landing. bad time of it. Every one feels like this sometime but the real question is do they really mean it? In my case of course, at that stage, I did not mean it. On reflection what I needed most and craved most was sleep. Long, deep, dissolving sleep. But I was not to get it immediately and not at all in the form I expected!

After some time he suggested that strong sleeping pills would help, but because in his view I was 'suicidal' these would have to be controlled and therefore I would have to agree to being admitted to hospital. I was so exhausted that the thought of a nice deep sleep in a comfortable hospital ward tended by a kind doctor and pretty nurses for a few days really appealed and I agreed to go. When my wife, a fully qualified nurse, was told she was greatly shocked and did her best to dissuade me. She had first hand experience of these places and just knew they were not at all right for my present condition, but I insisted, convinced that it would bring me rest. I could not have been more wrong!

The psychiatric wing of the hospital at first sight seemed ok but then it was viewed from my slumped position in my wheel chair but the reality of where I was did not register for some time as we went through endless questions about my state of mind. What has all this got to do with my exhaustion I thought, where are the sleeping pills and the comfy bed in a nice quiet side ward? Why were all these people dressed in tops and jeans, and the men with shaven heads, designer T shirts and Dock Marten's boots looking more like bouncers than male nurses? And the females, why did they sit on the floor with their clip board and questionnaire showing off their bare midriffs whilst stroking their long hair. What was all that about? What was a smartly suited middle aged man in shirt and tie to make of this charade?

And why this subtle (to them) constant innuendo of suicidal references. I just thank God I was sane enough to spot their little game and work my Obi-Wan-Kenobi trick of dodging it by waving my subliminal hand across their mind thus avoiding admitting to the 'S' word.

At last my wife reluctantly left me and I tried to settle in to this weird place. So still smartly dressed I began to give myself a conducted tour of the ward to see where the screams and moans where coming from, when I became aware that I was being closely watched. Spotting a comfy settee I sat down to read the newspaper laying there which disappointingly turned out to be a tabloid comic. Seeing the reaction, the observer silently, stealthily, slid into the next seat. Dressed conventionally and unusually wearing a full skirt, I thought she was a visitor. It was only after her more than passing interest in my life story and her attempt to guide me towards admitting the 'S' word that I rumbled her and started my own interrogation. Yep! Just as I suspected, a covert nurse in stealth mode. I might be in a lunatic asylum but I'm not daft! Looking disappointed she left empty handed.

Continuing my wander around the ward I casually came across a line diagram displayed on the wall and with growing unease I began to study it. It showed the progressive stages from admission to the thorough assessment to treatment to SECTIONING!

I had previously learnt the dreadful truth of this word in psycho speak when, because of his dysfunctional problems caused by the major brain damage, Andrew had been in a similar position and only my own efforts at the time had rescued him from the consequences of this diagnosis and had saved him. 'Sectioning' means you are assessed as being incapable of conducting your own affairs, you are considered a threat to yourself and others, and your liberty and freedom to operate as an individual are taken from you.

How I managed to remain composed and absorb the casual discovery of the gravity of my situation without panic or break down I do not know. This I DID know, my wife was right, I was in great danger and I had to somehow escape from this mad house.

I would have to play the next twenty four hours very carefully indeed.

Remarkably, despite my mental and physical exhaustion, I managed to quietly, even casually return to my bed space and in the next half an hour attempted to meditate reading first those words of truth about man's real nature that "the spirit in man is imperishable. Nothing can destroy the spirit. No, not even this depression I added."

It was then that my best friend Robert called to visit me. Boy was I glad to see him. What a stroke of good fortune this was. We could start to plan my escape, but first we needed somewhere secure to talk away from snooping eyes and ears of the Psyhco Police. So in an amazing recall of my characteristic manner, I adopted my sense of military self confidence and requested the use of the small staff conference room on the pretence of discussing my will. To my amazement they agreed. But only for half an hour!

Robert and I plotted quickly and quietly observed only by Iron Man (one of the macho shaven headed male nurses) in a black T shirt who glanced at us occasionally with suspicion as he walked by the glass walled conference room. The plot was that my wife Kathryn would persuade my GP that I had made a dreadful mistake in admitting myself to this asylum, and would return tomorrow with Robert and a family friend, Iain, who had been so helpful. Our GP was unwilling to come, but agreed to send a letter and answer any telephone query about my release.

Robert left before the search-light eyes of the patrolling watch tower guardian nurse Iron Man could catch him in the next suspicious sweep. I prepared for the night ahead and asked for a coat hanger to hang up my clothes in my bedside locker. The request was met with a patronising smile and never did arrive.

Time like eternity passed until it was time for bed and lights out, but at least and at last I would receive the powerful sleeping pill that would send me into a deep sleep. Something I had not had for months and desperately needed. This is what I had subjected myself to this horror for. This real nightmare that now surrounded me in this ward of mental illness, the wild screams, the frantic towing and frowing of the patient across the room opposite me, the tirade of expletives from behind the closed doors of the side ward, the call of restraint from the nursing staff.

Finally I closed my eyes and that greatest restorative power of nature, sleep, began to relieve me of all my pain and took me over, carrying me into that other world of sub consciousness and into a universal care of which we know nothing. It is a strange phenomenon of sleep, you only know you have been in it when you come out of it, whether it is in the day or night of your existence.

The next morning I rose feeling something of the benefit of the sleeping pill, showered and dressed in my business suit. Remember, I told myself, today is the great escape, so fight off the effects of the depression long enough to convince them you are ok; it had all been a great mistake, I'm not mad , I just need deep rest.

I packed my bags and after breakfast confidently told the office staff I would be 'checking out' once my friends had arrived later. They smiled in a condescending sort of way rather like a parent patronises a child asking for something that is forbidden. "We shall have to ask Doctor", they said, "she will see you soon".

Soon seemed for ever but finally Doctor Death and Iron Man nurse (as I named them) ushered me into the staff conference room and began the 'good cop, bad cop' interrogation routine. I was warned that anything I said would be used for my 'treatment'. "Remember we have the power to Section you" they said in a chilling almost sinister way. Good Lord, I was a step away from a padded locked cell! I was fighting for my life and this had to be the greatest performance of it! The effects of the fatigue caused by the depression gathered like storm clouds in my mind as I struggled to ward off any appearance of instability rather like an aircraft undergoes just before the stall. You know: nose high attitude; lowering air speed; reduction in noise level; ineffective controls. The telltale airframe buffet which heralds 'departure', the sickening plunge earthwards, the induced spin, the return to Sender would inexorably follow.

I would become 'detained' on their say so. I would loose instantly all my personal freedom. I would be at their mercy. Their cold blooded statement "We have the power to deny your release if we judge you to be mentally incapable" rang all the warning klaxons in my cockpit as I searched for the ejection seat handle.

In the most confident pose and prose I could muster, I carefully answered the cross examination under the intense armour piercing gaze of her small deep brown eyes and his right angular view slightly out of my peripheral vision somewhere in my four o'clock, his radar searching for any deviation or hesitation of my flight plan.

Good Lord I thought, these bandits are good, they had practised this before; they were certainly incoming and hostile! Mayday, Mayday!

Miraculously I remembered one of the practices I had learnt as a student of a Practical Philosophy course I had attended: come into the moment, feel your feet on the ground, be aware of all around you and give your full attention to what is before you.

I had used this before in other emergencies, it would surely not fail me now.

The interrogation lasted about an hour and at the end the doctor and nurse decided to postpone their judgement and left me to dwell upon it. It was then I just knew I had to forego any further offer of their hospitality! It was time to go JF; time for the great escape. I played for time whilst the guards were attending a meeting in another part of the hospital, then rang Kathryn and asked her to return with the letter from my GP and accompanied by our friend Iain.

With all the confidence I could muster I went to the office and told them that my wife had arrived with a note from my GP and we were ready to go home. 'Ah well your interview team are out at the moment, could you wait in the in ward café whilst we try to contact them about your leaving'? We did as asked and there then followed what seemed an eternity. The Staff Nurse returned saying he could not find them but was satisfied that all our papers were in order and we could cross the border (between sanity and insanity).

Trying not to run we did a fast taxi out of the special unit hoping we would not bump into the Inquisitors on the main runway. The getaway car was parked near by; the escape was complete! The first real battle was over but back home the real battle for survival from this deadly illness was about to begin.

As Churchill once said 'the battle of France is over; the Battle of Britain is about to begin. Upon it will depend the future of western civilisation and the freedom of our people. But if we fail all shall be cast into the abyss of darkness for a thousand years'.

Now the real darkness was to fall.

8   THE DARKEST HOUR

The darkest hour begins with the setting of the sun of belief in oneself; then come the clouds of confusion in the mind; then the forming of the ice on my wings that then could not lift me; the panic attacks; the growing nervousness, lack of confidence, self criticism, an unwillingness to engage in activity with or for others, fear of initiating anything new, a desire to go inside, to hide, to sleep, to pray it will all end. "Please God, make it all go away, let it end" screamed my mind!

The endless tossing and turning in bed made it impossible for my wife to sleep with me, so she moved into the front bedroom. The separation process had begun; the decent from a once happy marriage had commenced; the decline in all that was good and enjoyable inexorably followed. Hell was here; the great depression had begun.

For those who have fortunately never experienced deep depression it must be difficult to understand what it is like in there, and so, people say unhelpful things like, "oh! pull yourself together, snap out of it, get a grip! Well I'm here to tell you, if you could, you bloody well would!

It is blackness itself. Disease of the body, darkest day of the mind, the night of the soul, the loss of the spirit, the utter depth of hell.

During the darkest period of the depression, Kathryn my wife found that it was most helpful to share the problem with our close friend Margaret, wife of my best friend Robert and nightly texts were a feature of life and survival at that point. It didn't seem to matter what was said as long as there was a line of communication with another human being who was able to be on the outside of all of this nightmare.

The pair of them would send the most unlikely humorous messages in order to engage Kathryn's mind in anything other than the dreadful reality of the situation. They would exchange messages in the weirdest fashion, often with sentences without spaces between the words essentially to save money but which turned out to be so funny in attempting to decipher. The texts would often be encrypted in a Lancashire dialect, occasionally in Rupert Bear rhyme, and made the whole affair even more theatrical and bizarre.

OBSERVATION 1 :- KATHRYN FARRON

One thing that JF omits to mention (being too much of a gentleman really) is what I feel to be my own part in the lead up to his depression.

Around the time of Farnborough Air Show and the many other projects that John had on the go at that time, I was menopausal, suffering great mood swings and not a lot of fun to live with. Whilst he was trying to deal with his own illness and decrease in his usual level of confidence, he was also having to cope with a wife who MAY greet him with a smile as he came through the door, but equally likely may be lying in wait, rolling pin in hand, volume turned decidedly UP! Or possibly even worse than that could simply be quite morose with no explanation to give as to what the problem was.

Looking back now on that very difficult time, I realise that I was completely unaware (certainly in the beginning anyway) of the changes in him and never really took seriously his expressions of feeling a lack of confidence in himself or of his ability to complete a project. He ALWAYS completed projects for goodness sake, and they were always first class, so why didn't he just get on with it. I had much bigger things to worry about. 'I gained two pounds and fifteen more wrinkles this morning and he wants to talk about tickets not arriving for Farnborough Air Show' !!!!

Anyway, it was a tricky time all round and like most things in life there are usually many factors involved when the body becomes ill, whether it be physical or psychological illness, and indeed I believe the two to be intrinsically interlinked. So much so that I deem beyond any doubt that this element had some bearing on John's rapid decline once the illness got hold. By this time he had passed the point of no return and was desperately in need of help and I was shocked beyond belief to receive a call from our GP to say that John was collapsed in the surgery and about to be admitted to the Psychiatric Ward of our local hospital. The rest as they say is history ....

OBSERVATION 2 :- ROBERT MCNEILL (MY BEST MAN)

At first I just simply didn't believe it. Surely John was feigning it all and dramatising for effect. He's so confident and popular there was no way he could not face a stroll down the road to the local pond. But then there was the perspiring, the shaking, the hesitancy. What was going on there? This was not make-believe; he really was suffering.

And then there were his concerns about his work. The Air Pageant was heading for disaster. It would make the national head-lines. John had really screwed it up this time by not arranging for the aircraft to be there. He really believed there would be a head-line "Farnborough cancelled due to lack of aircraft. Squadron Leader Farron entirely to blame!"

Slowly, it began to dawn that this wasn't the John I knew. Someone else had assumed control as it were and the real John seemed absent. But, I couldn't accept that the John I knew had disappeared altogether; for some reason he had decided to hide under the covers (literally and psychologically!). We seemed to walk together to a foreign land at times and it was very dark. There was a light however – it was the light of consciousness conveyed through conversation. We had some wonderfully enlightening conversations and even though John immediately returned to the darkness on my leaving he nevertheless responded to my presence at the time.

Gradually, ever so gradually, the light got brighter or more accurately, the covers began to come off the light which was always there anyway. The first signs were the jokes at our own expense. We spent many an hour laughing heartily at this apparent great charade and it was inconceivable that recovery was not far away.

Two things stand out for me in all of this. Firstly, the illness was real, that the victim was really suffering; this needed acknowledging by friends and family. Secondly, the real "I" of the sufferer never leaves altogether but he does need reminding of his true stature, frequently.

This is where friends and family have a key role to play. To believe that the person we love has disappeared altogether is to believe the same untruths as the sufferer and our most useful role is to never forget that the real person behind all this is still present. That will never disappear.

OBSERVATION 3 :- MICHAEL CRANNY

John has lived in "interesting times". Whilst some of us have been coping with our ups and downs, John has been waiting for the next wave to hit him.

It has been that way for as long as I have known him. A life punctuated by challenges.

I am relieved I haven't had to face what he has.

I am glad my life has not been so "interesting"

In this book John describes how what we call "depression" has black-dogged him.

I am sure I don't really know what depression is, what causes it, or what cures it, but I do know that escape is possible, and I hope by reading this book you will agree.

There is hope. The hope is already in the tunnel with you. It is that tiny light, shining the in darkness that surrounds you.

It is you.

You have to keep it alight.

Medicine helps, friendship helps, and as John has found, philosophy – trying to know yourself, also helps.

The whole point of this book is to say that there is always HOPE, and provided you turn to it, it will work for you. In that respect John did nothing. Hope did it all.

Since John came out of the tunnel, he has faced a multiple heart bypass as well as a mid-air collision, and his revived business is now involved in a project involving both the UK and the South African air forces, so nothing changes and he soldiers on, fighting one battle after another.

There is one quotation I have always found useful – it is from the Bhagavad-Gita

"This inner severance from the affliction of misery is spirituality.

It should be practised with determination

and with a heart which refuses to be depressed."

If depression comes your way, run in the opposite direction, and if you can, just refuse to have anything to do with it.

The important point to make here is the absolute necessity for those close to the patient to have recourse to some understanding person who is able to view the situation objectively from a complete outsider's point of view, thus providing the essential detachment that is necessary to maintain one's sanity.

The outside observer is able to assist the insider by constantly reminding them of the memory of the patient's true qualities and personality. This memory is vital in sustaining truth about the patient and is used to overcome the dreadful persistence of the denial by the patient which constantly reinforces the condition and is therefore extremely painful for close family to cope with.

There is this awful dichotomy of watching all one's powers of self respect slip away from you whilst knowing you are somehow helpless to stop it. This is terrifying. At this stage the effect of the depression is a slow progression and ratchets itself up in increments determined by what the mind perceives as a threat or a problem.

This threat can appear in all sorts of ways and is not a respecter of rank or status as I discovered on January 1st 2001 when I received a letter from the Duke of Edinburgh telling me that I had been appointed MBE in the Queen's New Years Hours list.

There was no jubilation, no joy at receiving such an honour, all sense of happiness that one might expect to naturally arise was swamped in a cold dread that I would need to go to the Palace and face the Queen.

I promptly hid the historic communiqué in great fear of its consequences.

The citation read : To Our trusty and well beloved John Farron, Squadron Leader in Our Royal Air Force Reserve for unstinting service in the field of Air Training etc, etc,…. and I hid it away!

Although it does appear as a single act of refusing to accept the truth about the condition, you know, that it is an illness. In fact what I observed was that, in order to exist at all, the conditioning of one's mind to accept the effects of depression, there is a highly active sub conscious computer-like process activity that repeatedly denies the truth about one's self. That is, that one is the observer of what is going on in the mind, not the though processes which are being observed.

This all happens behind the surface of the mind that is normally apparent. To take yet another aeronautical analogy - modern fast jet fighter aircraft are designed to be unstable to enable 'high alpha – angle of attack' and therefore high manoeuvrability in dog fights. To control this, a computer manages an ultra high rate of control inputs, micro second by micro second, to prevent the aircraft from departing from its flight path or going out of control.

In depression the process works in reverse. The mind continually maintains the instability.

Clever isn't it?

Now if only there where something faster than the mind?

An ancient book of wisdom, the Eesha Upanishads says: The Self is one. Unmoving, it moves faster than the mind. The senses lag, but Self runs ahead. Unmoving, it out runs pursuit. Out of Self comes the breath that is the life of all things.

So, what ever is observing the mind is clearly faster than the mind, ergo it could interrupt the conditioning process previously mentioned in the analogy.

If only we knew that and could introduce the separation necessary to deal with the cause of the problem of total identification with the belief that - I am - the depression. Because, how can you be that which you can observe? There is you and there is it!

Of course it is easy now upon reflection for me to spell it out so simply. At the time it was not so. One should not under estimate the strength of this dis-ease of the mind. It is enormously and almost all pervasive, being as it is powered by your own consciousness.

At the time it is pretty dire. How I got through those darkening days and on 13March 2001 faced up to the trial of going to receive the MBE from Her Majesty in person, and in front of all those people, I shall never know.

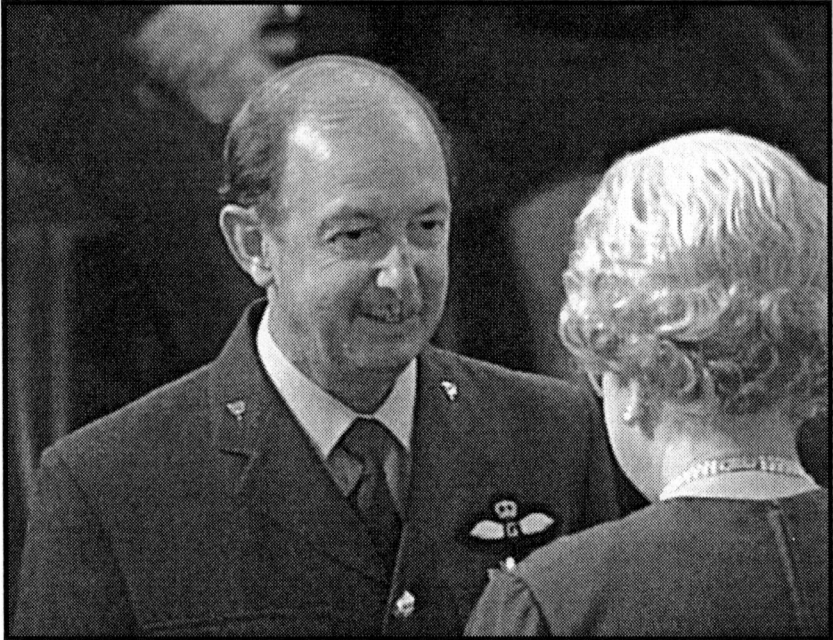

THE STRAIN SHOWS!
MEETING THE QUEEN
MARCH 2001

From then on things got steadily worse.

I became more and more of a recluse hiding in my bedroom which became my prison cell to which only I had the key. I refused to go out or answer the door, or telephone, or correspondence. I wilfully cut myself off from all my family and friends. Only the most determined like Iain, Robert and Michael were not deterred. They would constantly visit me in my self imposed prison encouraging me to wash, bathe and shave, all essential personal care I was no longer interested in.

Robert would ring every day. "Hello John. Are you there? Pick up the phone John. John pick up the phone lets just chat. Shall I call round to see you tonight? Pick up the phone John, go on mate, let's talk". "Fancy a pint John?"

I rarely did, but he never gave up. This tenacious bloody New Zealander terrier never gave up. For that I owe him one of my many lives. On the battle field of life you need real heroes like Robert McNeill. If I was ever to go to war I would want to fly with real men like him as my wing man. A truly Best Man and for all seasons.

'The friends thou hast and their adoption tried, grapple them to thy self with hoops of steel' said Polonius in his advice to his son in Hamlet. In deepest depression, you need real friends to believe in you, who never forget you, who hold the truth about you, who act as your memory until you awake again to your former self. This is the most important thing family and friends can do for anyone suffering in this way.

Their persistence along with my flying colleagues at the Squadron helped to restore me to life. Another of my personal rescue team who is to be mentioned in despatches is Michael Cranny. An unlikely character for sympathetic mollycoddling any one, let alone his friend Biggles, locked as he was in this aerial dog fight for his life.

His objective, incisive, tenacious, cool and calculating intellect combined with a wicked wit would find tiny holes in my solid armour of thick torpor. His use of black humour matched my own causing me to return fire in a brilliantly calculated strategy to draw me out in to the open field of banter battle. An engagement he knew only to well I could not resist. In the past we had often fought with friendly fire crossing our swords to cut through the absurdities of life. To day he was out to save mine.

His favourite device was the letter, and with his permission I reprint one of them here:

Stockport, Cheshire 15 January 2002

Dear John,

You are our test case and if we fail you, we fail ourselves, so please start humming to a new sound, one that will lead you out of the depths and back into life and stop lying to yourself.

You are Great, you are Immortal, Glorious and the Support of all. The lies you have told yourself are only lies. They only cover what is true. They change nothing.

If you need help, help will be provided. If you need hope it will appear from the bottom of Pandora's box, where you now languish. But if you want to be left alone, forget it. This option is not an option.

You remember Pathos – well you are in it, and you remember that to get out of it you need help from the outside. You can't pull yourself up by your own bootstraps.

You need help.

I am no expert at depression, although I have in error often courted her, and I know she fancies me. I am not the one to give you advice, but I am good at guessing, and I guess that a good start would be with medication.

Be brave and take the happy pills.

They will work, they will alleviate the state, they will not cure you, but they would be a good place to re-start.

It wouldn't take much effort would it to put your daft arguments down and follow medical advice, it can't be any worse than what you are doing to us all now.

You could also telephone me, Yes! you could telephone me!
Now wouldn't that be nice?

Your best friend
Michael

So at last I took Michael's advice and agreed to take the pills which although they took weeks to begin to work, did eventually have some effect and at least mitigated the worst far edges of the depression, a sort of damping effect. You know like in aerodynamics when the effects of flutter in the wings is controlled by adjusting structural airframe stiffness and the harmonic frequencies of vibration generated with increased velocity, that sort of thing. Just like the mind in high frequency it needs a damper to reduce excessive agitation.

Michael also persuaded me to seek help from a Consultant Psychiatrist called Dr. Patel who was highly recommended by my GP.

And so, one very dark winter's night Dr. Patel came to the house accompanied by Michael, Kathryn and my GP. It was agreed that Dr. Patel and I would meet down stairs whilst every one else huddled together around a single bar electric fire in the upstairs study, that was until we had a power cut and we all resorted to 'ill met by candle light'.

However, how absurd it all seems now, it does show the lengths to which friends and family were prepared to go to save me. Never give up hope!

I never had any faith in psychiatrists until I met Dr. P in that candle lit encounter and subsequent appointments with him proved just how wrong you can be about seeking help with depression. He was a man of immense patience and understanding and he never tried to psycho analyse me or super impose any theory on me. He knew I would not accept that.

Dr. Patel mostly just listened, but with FULL attention.

At each appointment I would insist on Robert, Michael, Ian or Kathryn accompanying me to ensure I was not tempted to lie and to tell the truth as accurately as possible. This is an important lesson. Truth and admission of one's condition is vital to the healing process. It worked like this.

My escort team, as I called them, would provide factual reminders as to my true character; that I was a man of action, highly intelligent, articulate, courageous, ambitious, a natural leader, a very strong man with compassion for others and great love for his family. Some one who would stand and fight for what was right and true, who was brave and a real survivor and had endurance, patience and fortitude.

Not this apparent wretched wreck we see before us.

This is the vital role those who support must provide. A memory in locum parenthesis.

By now I would wake up each morning with the immediate feeling of total hopelessness, self criticism and hate in the unhealthiest state of body, mind, and nature. That was my entire existence, except for one very powerful desire - to kill myself.

Each day I would plan how to do it, to top myself. There were many and varied ways. I was ready to bale out, to cut the parachute cords of this life.

Why did I not do it? Who really knows? This I did know; I just had to hang on in there; ABOVE ALL...HANG ON! Somehow I had to survive, to endure, to recover control of this badly damaged soul in this perilous flight. I used every device I could think of including sounding the mantra for the system of meditation I had been given some many years earlier. At the time it seemed ineffective, but on reflection I believe it did help to prevent the worse.

I would toss and turn in and on my bed wrestling with an invisible demon in sheer frustration at my condition. Out of the depths I have cried to thee, Oh Lord, Lord hear my voice! It could not be done alone. I needed help. At last I had admitted that it was an illness.

This is a most important stage in the whole awful business; to admit that depression is an illness and seek help.

The admission that I needed help, that this was a serious illness, had finally stopped me from denying the truth.

However things were to get much worse, much worse. I started to drink steadily until I had emptied the well stocked drinks cabinet and was consuming several bottles of wine each day thereafter. I became in my view an alcoholic, but it is interesting that in a perverse way this helped the suffering and probably helped to weaken the will to die.

Then came the darkest hour; the blackest moment; the cruellest time of this tragic tale. In a fit of combined frustration, sheer desperation and blind rage, I threw Kathryn and James out onto the street! Thank God without physical violence, but with terrible verbal abuse. I told her to get out! Shouting abuse as she fled up the street in shock and utter disbelief. How had it come to this? How could I? What demon had NOW possessed me?

Fortunately she was able to fly to our friends Robert and Margaret and then later to another close friend of ours, Mary Swindlehurst, who took in both of them in an expression of sheer generosity which was so characteristic of this lady's magnanimity. Here they would be safe from harm. Here they would shelter from the tempest raging in my mind. But for me the anger fuelled storm would rage on and on and on.

As the Bard would say; "how fortunate are we in the friends we have and their adoption tried."

From then on I would confine myself to the upstairs study over looking the Withnell Forrest from where this tale began and, rather like the decent in to the Dark Ages, draw a heavy curtain of blackness over all my worlds. This thick blackness seeped in to the walls, the carpets, the curtains, the furniture, the bedding, the clothes and especially the old dressing gown I wore constantly. A gross form of protective blanket I would wrap around my self to ward off the effects of good company my friends and family could provide.

Without doubt good company is essential to the recovery from depression as I was about to come to understand first hand.

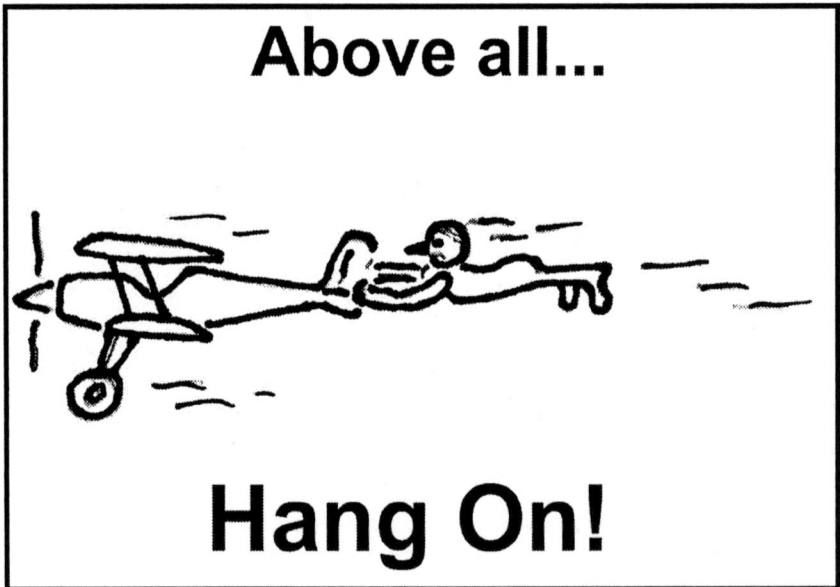

Above all...

Hang On!

9 THE ABC OF D FOR DEPRESSION

One of the strange conditions of my recovery from deep depression was the step to participating in a sort of black humour. It is a game of the mind in which you in some way start to re-engage with the world around you by laughing at or your perceived condition. It is a sort of self deprecation process in which you start to put distance between the other wise firm belief that you are all those doubts about your self which form the basis of the depression and which so firmly binds you; your own worst enemy. It is a very first step "outside" and as such is of major importance. This is the form in which it came:

1ST MAY 2003

Dawn has broken on this dreadful subterranean world of depression and thank God there is a chink of light as the jaws of this vice allows the mind to force open its grip with an attempt at humour – black humour. I start to attack the pathos of my situation by mocking the condition and getting the vital space of separation between me and the total identification with this deep chasm of illness called 'depression'. Miraculously I start to want, however feebly, to fight back. To cast off this 'shameful despondency' as Krishna once said to Arjuna in the wisdom of the Geeta. To use this sleeping sword in my hand and build a new Jerusalem in these green and pleasant lands that truly surround

71

me. Enough of the dark satanic mills in the deep, deep shafts of the mind, I choose life not death, I choose light not darkness, I choose life not death – its war!

Look now it's the 1st of May.

Mayday, Mayday, Mayday!

Mayday, as you all know is the international distress call for all in peril.

And it's time to spell out the message to mock this condition:

D is for Depression and all who Dwell in or perish in her.

D is also for Determined to be Depressed and be Devoted to it.

Honours can be won here e.g.

D is for Distinguished Order of Depression (DoD); can also be pronounced 'Dead on Delivery'

D is for Denial of the d' whole thing.

Depression is not for Dorks. It is a very serious condition of despondency in the Deep Blue/Blackness of ones' soul mate - Ego!

D is for Doom – even to the edge of it; go on, you can get closer, even closer, teeter on the edge.

D is for Demise. Oh! Poor Me! I am so helpless, poor, poor me.

D is for Disgrace as in (Shakespeare's sonnet 29 – 'When in Disgrace with Fortune and men's eyes, I alone beweepe my out-cast state, and trouble deafe heaven with my bootlesse cries, and looke upon myself and curse my fate') an essential condition to be depressed.

D is also for de Teenager – a natural form of adolescent depression, appears in both sexes. Sex like all other drugs leads to depression – often through the lack of it!

D is for Different types of Depression as follows:

Menu   -   1) Metrological Depression

2) Geographical Depression

3) Clinical Depression

3) Manic Depression

5) Deep Depression

E is for Ego …..

Ego is essential to a successful depression. Without it there would be no-one to be able to feel the angst, the hurt, the tragedy, the pain, the sorrow, the ME of it all.

E is for Eyes. I went out to buy a pair of reading glasses recently but got Depressed because I could not read the telephone number of the Opticians, bus time table, fare information OR my prescription.

E is for Extension of Excruciation of the need for pain – after all it's my Depression and I'll be sad if I want to; cry if I want to; be damned if I want to, be depressed if I want to. Readers can sing along in tune with a melancholic refrain sung on a rainy Monday morning while listening to the Carpenters:- 'Mondays always get me down'.

E is also for Environmental Depression, so necessary in keeping the right conditions for being under-the-weather. eg. Cyclonic Depression – a low point (cold front) of atmospheric pressure designed to fill an undesirable region of a high anti-cyclonic pressure system associated with a warm front; bright sunshine, a good-to-be-alive-happy-days-are-here-again, and such other unwelcome feelings which can dangerously come close to raising your mood and destroying your depression.

E is for Egocentricity which is vital for self centred subjective consideration dwelling on ME, ME, ME. On no account should this micro cosmic concern for ME be allowed to expand to reach out to others or anything else that might lift one's mood.

E is also for Epidemic. Britain is in the grip of an epidemic of Depression. It is estimated that one sixth of the population suffer from the disease at a cost to the taxpayer of 7 billion pounds.

P is for the Parrot on your shoulder, re-affirming all that's wrong with you. It feeds

on seeds of doubt and nags incessantly.

"What a pretty mess, what a pretty mess, eh? eh? pretty mess?

P "is for Pressure, Panic, Pain, and Pessimism.

Please, Displease ME, oh yeah, like I Displease you !

Plan ahead for topping yourself – you know how. How many times have you said it – go on, this is your unlucky day, sink to the occasion, treat yourself – you've earned it.

P is also for hacked off! The more the better, get really – hacked off – yes really! So hacked off I am with me, you, him, her, them, us, it, that, also others I cannot think of because I'm really hacked off.

P is for Past – dwell in it, roll in it, play it, live it, relish it, never get past it, over it, out-of-it or forget it. Never be present, this will displace the depression – watch out for the tell-tale signs – awareness, seeing, smelling, touching, tasting, hearing – these lead you into the light of reality and away from your beloved darkness and despair which can only exist in the past or in a projection of the imagined future. A world wholly created for me and my suffering – depressing isn't it?

P is also for Pathos – no, not a Greek tragedy but a real disturbed state. Repeated doses of loss of ones attention to a 'captured' condition leads to loss of awareness – pathos – Depression.

R is for Regression, a vital tactic to counter any sign of improvement – not to be confused with R for Recovery or Rehabilitation.

R is for ready to admit defeat, resignation, resistance to help, cure, comfort, regeneration or recovery.

R is for remission. OED: forgiveness of sins; remitting of debt, penalty etc

R is for repeating circling thoughts of worthlessness, self pity, hopelessness, unhappiness, death without glory, inner conversations with the ventriloquist's dummy in the head, negative thoughts, which circle for all eternity in your mind keeping out dangerous good or cheering ideas which might creep in, should you pause for a moment and remember your real self.

Worse still, do not come into the moment now; the present condition of just being. The parrot in your head or on your shoulder will remind you of it – the dualistic nature of your ego – the real cause of your depression. Listen to the parrot, he or she is the master of all argument about who you really are and convince you of the lie that you are not what you really are in truth – Your True Self!

E is for Endless misery which is the result of ignoring who I really am and insisting on being all those things that I believe I am not. In truth you cannot be what you observe since you are the observer and not the object of observation. (See diagram as follows :)

OBJECTIVITY TEST

Observer ——————⟶ Object

(Me)   (That)

QED You cannot be that which you observe!

No! Not even This Depression!

This realisation that one is not what one observes leads to separation from it!

But hey! If you want misery, ignore this truth and please forgive me for bringing it to your observation.

Fact – you cannot be what you observe, no matter how holy or how horrible!

E is for expectations – be careful here, this just might lift the gloom through a process of hope, an effective and little used natural feeling which can induce a probability of improvements or decline in depression. This leads to aspirations which, if repeated could decrease the darkness encasing the soul and lift your mood.

E is a vowel which can also express an exclamation of wonder, delight, brightness and other dangerous conditions. For example, Ee lad! Ee by gum, E int it grand up North !

S stands for sleep – oh! that much desired condition, so much sought after to assist the depression to receive regular maintenance through many doses and by any means. For example, natural, medication induced, boredom, drink, watching old films (especially morose), sentimental, sad, melancholic, or say by visiting the Tate Modern's gallery of darkness.

S stands for sure of sadness, simulation of any remorseful act from the past on which one can dwell or escape the present and which might contain an opportunity for a lift of mood or aspect.

S is of course for suicide, you know the 'biggy', the ultimate self destruct weapon, the way to end it all – that is until the next rebirth anyway. Repeated doses of this will no doubt have an effect upon your Brownie Points for future embodiments and the allocation of consciousness necessary to continue ones journey through the universe as a human being. Ah! 'To be or not to be'. That really is the question. I guess if you are not 'being' then you are not – well, anything or maybe worse, something of lower or less consciousness – say a donkey or a brick.

S Also stands for sin! Now we are talking the real stuff of (especially western) guilt complexes. Mea culpa, mea culpa, Mea Maxima culpa. Go for it. You know - It's your fault, you are to blame. Like they say, the Ego must prevail, if it cannot be right, it most certainly will be wrong. Yes go on, be to blame.

I is for I as in I am. This personal pronoun, I the Self or the ego. The subject or object of self consciousness is a double edged sword of truth and denial. So watch it! It can cut either way. For example, you can believe, I am the depressing thoughts about myself, or that the pronoun could be used to say, I am – great, happy, alive, wonderful, simply the best, not all this other stuff that I imagine I am, you know – small, unhappy, dead, hopeless, simply awful.

I, of course is for ignorance. Now we're getting down to it. This simple but deadly effective act is a real all-in-one tool. Multi faceted in its effect it comes as second nature to most people. I mean, look around, people do it all the time: ignoring the reality of the wonder of creation and themselves; choosing to be bothered rather than bright; selecting sadness rather than sunlight; dwelling in the dark rather than shining in the sunlight of their own Self; living a lifeless existence fed on the poverty of the mind of their choice. I should know, I have practised it for long enough.

I can't, won't, I shan't, I could not possibly, are all useful negative terms for sustaining depression and repetition of these will ensure you stay well and, of course, truly depressed!

I can't see the point of it all; Life, love, mankind, the creation, the universe. Be careful here, do not disturb this introspection with dangerous reminders of the Truth such as Shakespeare's Sonnet 33 ....

> *Full many a glorious morning have I seene,*
>
> *Flatter the mountaine tops with soveraine eie,*
>
> *Kissing with golden face the meadows greene;*
>
> *Guilding pale streames with heavenly alcumy:*
>
> *Anon permit the basest cloudes to ride,*
>
> *With ougly rack on his cellestiall face,*
>
> *And from the for-lorne world his visage hide*
>
> *Stealing unseene to west with this disgrace:*
>
> *Even so my Sunne one early morne did shine,*
>
> *With all triuimphant splendor on my brow,*
>
> *But alack, he was but one houre mine,*
>
> *The region cloude hath mask'd him from me now.*
>
> *Yet him for this, my love no whit disdaineth,*
>
> *Suns of the world may staine, whe heavens sun stainteh.*
>
> *Note how quickly the dark clouds can return unless one is vigilant.*

O is for 'Only Me'. I am unique in this condition and only Me has this problem. Of course this is self sustaining and axiomatic, causing a grain of truth to emerge in the brief but powerful reinforcement of the conditioning process of the mind. Ah yes! Only Me could be like this. Nobody understands Me! Yes, depression is a little understood and damming condition causing great suffering. All joking aside, whatever can be done to educate people in general about this illness should be done.

Education should start with teaching people the truth about themselves through the process of self discovery. Guide them towards the gradual awareness of their own Being. Remember, that which is in presence cannot be denied. Help them to practise the simple exercise of awareness, to live in the moment, the present continuous wherein lays happiness, knowledge and bliss.

Perhaps we could try an experiment. Try this at home folks:

THE EXERCISE

First, sit quietly and let go of any tensions, physical or mental...

Let the mind fall still....

Be aware of being present, here and now...

Feel the touch of your feet on the ground ...

The weight of the body on the chair ...

Feel the touch of the clothes on the skin ...

And the play of air on the face and hands ...

If they are open, let the eyes receive colour and form without comment ...

Taste ...

Smell ...

Be fully here ...

Now be aware of hearing ...

Let sounds be received and let them come and go without comment or judgment of any kind ...

With the body completely relaxed, let the hearing run right out to the furthest sounds, and to the stillness beyond...

Simply rest in this great awareness of stillness for a few moments... rest... just rest.

N is for negativity, the denial, the negation of all that is true about one's nature and the indulging of all that is untrue. This is perhaps the greatest tool of depression, the terrible power to set all things at nought. The creation of a living hell of denial of one's true nature, knowledge, happiness and the means to enjoy it in bliss for ever. Even a small appreciation of this fundamental truth about one's being is enjoyable, fulfilling and satisfying.

N is for not knowing or ignoring the truth about oneself, which is the same in all creatures. 'A man who sees Himself in himself and Himself in all other creatures knows no sorrow'. Ancient Upanishad wisdom.

Imagine – knows NO sorrow.

N is for not being and deliberately trying to be something, anything else, anything other than one's self which always exists in the moment now and is happy always.

Watch the mind! Watch in particular the movements of the mind. Watch THINKING. Thinking is particularly useful in destroying your life – so think about it.

Here is a wonderful analogy given to me by Michael Cranny. Its source is unknown but I am indebted to its author:

IS THINKING DESTROYING YOUR LIFE ?

It started out innocently enough. I began to think at parties now and then to loosen up. Inevitably though, one thought led to another, and soon I was more than just a social thinker.

I began to think alone – "to relax" I told myself – but knew it wasn't true. Thinking became more and more important to me, and finally I was thinking all the time.

I began to think on the job. I knew that thinking and employment don't mix, but I couldn't stop myself. I began to avoid friends at lunchtime so I could read Thoreau and Kafka.

I would return to the office dizzied and confused, asking,

"What is it exactly we are doing here?" Things weren't going so great at home either. One evening I had turned off the TV and asked my wife about the meaning of life. She spent that night at her mother's.

I soon had a reputation as a heavy thinker. One day the boss called me in. He said, "Skippy, I like you and it hurts me to say this, but your thinking has become a real problem. If you don't stop thinking on the job, you'll have to find another job". This gave me a lot to think about.

I came home early after my conversation with the boss. "Honey," I confessed, "I've been thinking ...."

"I know you've been thinking," she said, "and I want a divorce!"

"But Honey, surely it's not that serious".

"It is serious," she said, lower lip quivering. "You think as much as college professors and college professors don't make any money, so if you keep on thinking we won't have any money!"

"That's faulty logic" I said impatiently, and she began to cry. I'd had enough. "I'm going to the library," I snarled as I stomped out the door.

I headed for the library, in the mood for some Nietzsche, with NPR on the radio. I roared into the parking lot and ran up to the big glass doors ... they didn't open. The library was closed.

To this day, I believe that a Higher Power was looking out for me that night.

As I sank to the ground clawing at the unfeeling glass, whimpering for Zarathustra, a poster caught my eye. "Friend, is heavy thinking ruining your life?" it asked. You probably recognize that line. It comes from the standard Thinker's Anonymous poster.

Which is why I am what I am today: a recovering thinker. I never miss a TA meeting. At each of these meetings we watch a non-educational video; last week it was "Porky's". Then we share experiences about how we avoided thinking since the last meeting.

I still have my job, and things are a lot better at home. Life just seemed …. easier somehow, as soon as I stopped thinking.

STOP THINKING AND ENJOY YOURSELF!

So there you have it, ten letters that spell out possibly the most dreadful, feared and destructive word in our vocabulary and one of the prime precursors of leading to it-thinking.

Depression, a condition of mind, body and soul, an illness about which little is known but which is crippling the western world, and if you suffer from depression, you are, sadly, far from being alone. In fact, it has been estimated that there may be over 300 million people in the world today who suffer from it.

Why is this? Why should this be the great plague of our time? Why should it be so common and widespread and left apparently so little understood?

Are we condemned to suffer this silent and deadly killer in ignorance, or should we really be able to take up arms against this black sea of troubles and by opposing end therein?

Remember – all things are fair in love and the war against depression. Whatever it takes. Take it, try it, test it. It is different for everyone, the key is action, movement of any kind is better than the terrible mal and torpor of the Black Dog as Churchill called it. Always remember it is an illness and if great people like Churchill and Alexander the Great can get it so can we lesser mortals. Accept that action, and that alone will bring about the separation from the curse of identification with the delusion which lies at the evil roots of attachment to depression.

Ah yes, attachment, now there's a thing! It seems we can attach ourselves to anything – yes anything. Any physical, mental or spiritual thing in or out of this universe. What a power, what an awesome capability, what surreal potential at our immediate disposal. Ready now at any moment simply by the act of claiming, for example – this is mine! That is mine! My life, my body, my mind, my soul, my job, my unemployment, my shirt, my car, my house, my land, my idea, my thoughts, my feelings, my party (and I'll cry if I want to), sigh if I want to, be depressed if I want to, die if I want to.

What an awesome choice we have, what extra ordinary ability to be or not to be, what a piece of work is Man!

Yes I want, I claim, I have. Thus we sentence ourselves. Observe how it works, note the grammar;

> I
>
> I am
>
> I am a man/woman
>
> I am a good/bad man/woman
>
> I am a bright/dull good/bad man/woman
>
> I am a happy/unhappy, bright/dull, good/bad man/woman
>> etc. etc.

And so the sentencing process goes on ad infinitum. But then! Then, comes the crunch. We start to believe it, we become attached to it, we are IT !

As a child I can recall this game of just being. Just being myself and how happy I was by nature, just so, not dependent on anything. Then one day along came this idea to pretend to be someone, some thing, some other. A great game I thought. I could be anything and know I was just playing at IT. I would watch the play and enjoy the fun. Then one day along came attachment to the toy, the part, the game. Then one day I forgot that it was my self just watching, observing, detached but enjoying the play. I forgot that it was I that was watching and I became identified with the object. I became IT! And so I became an identity, groomed it, pampered it, preserved it, nurtured it, made it my own and all that went with it. Was this better than the simple happiness of the child? Unlimited, free from fear, care, concern, by just being.

As the famous Bear of Little Brain, Winne-the-Pooh, points out, there are great dangers in thinking and of over use of the brain in trying to do the important things that it is not equipped for.

And a Bear of Little Brain should know!

A brain can do all kinds of things, but these are not necessarily the most important things. Abstract cleverness of mind only separates the thinker from the world of reality, because of too many, who think too much and care too little.

10 FROM DARKNESS TO LIGHT

The very first chinks of light in an otherwise desperately dark mind appeared shortly after the crucial decision to choose life rather than death. This came some three years after the start of the nervous break down which marked the entry into the major phase of the deep depression.

I awoke in the early hours of one morning in April 2003 and there it was, the question - do you want to live or die? It was as black and white as that and I knew it had to be one or the other.

I chose life.

This light appeared in the very simple the decision to move this sluggish body and involve it in some form, any form of physical activity such as making a cup of tea, washing up, or attempting any kind of movement. The vital step was to re-engage with the senses starting with the sense of sight in a very slight, but very slight, movement. Movement/ activity is THE key.

At first it was an enormous effort to bring the physical body to climb out of the pit of despair into which I had hidden it for so long. To just get out of bed required all the strength I could muster. I teetered on the edge willing with a weak and feeble mind this body - which once was so alive, fit and healthy, which once had won a Blue in athletics, captained swimming, soccer and tennis teams, climbed mountains, run cross-country, flown with the Red Arrows, raced yachts and flown many thousands of hours as a pilot in all kind of weather - to stand up and just take the first step out of the black night of the soul.

And so began the first flickering subtle flame of light to enter the being for nearly three years. How I cherished that moment of renaissance as I approached the kitchen sink and once again made a connection between the inert mind and the sense of touch. Once more I could observe the hands in the water washing the cups, just feeling the warmth of the water, just able to rest in the truth that I was not that which I could observe especially the beliefs in the mind that I was that depression. Once again the memory of what I was not had slowly but surely returned and I was again a human, just being.

It was at this early and fragile stage of the recovery that I discovered a simple trick in encouraging the process of action and essential movement. I had a photograph of my youngest son James on the windowsill showing him sitting back in an arm chair relaxed and smiling, sticking out his arms with his hands clenched in a thumbs up gesture of approval. This is just what I needed, his seeming approval of my effort tiny though it was from the father he once knew and loved. How I needed that love, that recognition.

I repeated this process of homily to the photograph each time I completed a task however small and it began to work its magic. Slowly, very slowly, I began, day by day, to gain enough strength physically and mentally to persevere.

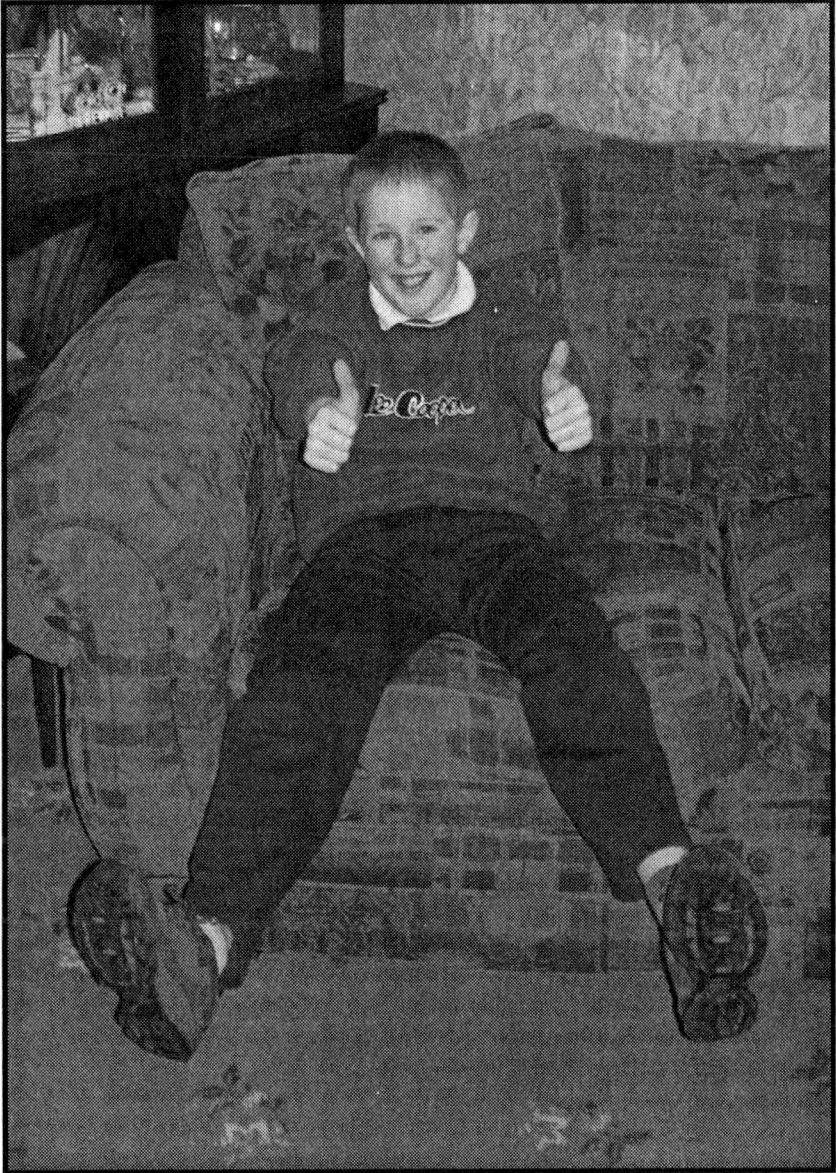

JAMES'S
GESTURE OF APPROVAL

Another useful device in restoring one's mind to health in the recovery phase is the use of a technique which I call the 'Short List'

Create a short, simple list of easily attainable tasks such as; wash cups; make bed; sweep yard; and write them down numbering them 1,2,3 etc. Then give your full attention to completing each simple job one at a time taking all the time you wish. No pressure and definitely no rush. As each one is done, tick off with great flourish because what you have achieved is proportionately quite a lot when compared to your previous state of near total immobility. Do not under estimate the effect this will have as you gradually move down the list ticking off your accomplishments.

This simple performance does several things:

1. It is something to look forward to - a sort of mission
2. It is a simple measure of achievement
3. It brings hope for the future
4. It lifts the heart
5. It helps to re habilitate the mind.

At this stage small steps are what is needed.

THE SHORT LIST

1   3 or 4 items
2   Simple tasks
3   Short duration
4   Easily achievable
5   No stresses
6   Engage the mind and senses
7   Enjoy the sense of achievement

Time in the recovery phase was marked with great caution as I carefully did a little more each day regaining the simple delights of cleanliness, proper dress and order. However I had still not ventured outside of the house for nearly two years even though the people in the village, who fortunately, unlike me had not lost their sense of humour, had constantly enquired of my son Andrew how Biggles was fettling? That is until one day Andrew, who had kept me alive during the darkest days of the depression with butties from the Top Shop, fish and chips from Elsie's chippy and endless pints from the Oak Tree pub, declared we had run out of food. He tactfully suggested that we go to Blackburn to buy some.

Unfit to drive through sheer muscle atrophy, I was very nervous about Blackburn. This would mean the bus, people, crowds! Andrew coaxed me out of the house heavily disguised to avoid recognition and therefore communication with villagers and neighbours. People would ask questions. "Where had I been for the last three years?" "What's bin up wi'thee lad?" Those sort of awkward questions I so desperately wanted to avoid.

Now the bus stops in the village are opposite each other, one going down to Blackburn and one going up to Chorley. The former has no shelter and I feared that waiting there would cause encounters with folk passing by, so I hid in the back of the shelter at the bus stop on the other side, telling Andrew to warn me of the approaching bus. Shortly people came to pass him by and enquired where he was going and who with? "Blackburn with mi' Dad" he replied. "And where's thi' Dad young Andrew"? "Oh he's hiding in yon bus shelter." " 'Allo Mister Farron", they chorused waving madly!

I tried to ignore them by burying myself deeper into the recesses when I was joined by a little old lady who enquired where I was going. "Blackburn" I grunted from behind my muffled scarf and aircrew sunglasses. "E lad, buzzes go to Chorley from 'ere, tha wants t'other side."

It was at that point that the ice on my wings began to melt. The sheer comicality of the situation and the cathartic effect of the warmth of this northern humour was so compelling that three years of case hardening of my heart against all comers, even this veteran miserable ego, could not resist it. So when the 'buz' came, Andrew and I sat up stairs on the front seats and giggled like a couple of kids all the way to Blackburn.

Other ventures out followed like the trip to visit the Squadron. My old pal and Chief Flying Instructor Alan Howard called at the house one day as he had done on many occasions before over the past three years. This time it was different. This time I let him in! Now CFI'S are never fazed and this surprise was no exception. "I thought you might like a ride out to the airfield, meet the chaps, enjoy the space, that sort of thing" he said in his characteristic casual matter-of-fact way. I hesitated, worrying about the thought of meeting my fellow flying instructors after such a long period of self imposed exile. What would they think? What would they say about my condition? How would they view this enigma of depression, something we did not discuss in the Mess. In military circles psychological problems are usually hedged around with awkward unease and generally not considered in service parlance. Fast planes, fast cars and fast w-workouts were more usual." Well, I said, maybe just for the ride. No crowd of welcome home types and certainly no aircraft"

We arrived at the Squadron to a warm but quiet welcome. Alan had obviously briefed the team and since it was a warmish day he and I sat on the casual chairs by the side of the air traffic control caravan just opposite the aircraft dispersal. "Gerry's late again" joked Alan, scanning the empty sky. (A reference to the way RAF pilots used to anticipate Luftwaffe attacks during the Battle of Britain.)

Just then an aircraft landed and taxied into Dispersal. Shutdown checks complete, the canopy opened and out jumped Flight Lieutenant Ian Taylor my former 'wing man' and old buddy. "Hi JF, great to see you. The weather's crap for teaching students but its OK for seasoned pilots like you. Fancy a spot of SCT?" "You are joking. You won't get me back in the air again" I replied "and anyway I haven't got my flying suit with me". "That's OK" chirped Alan, "you can use my spare, I just happen to have it with me". I was beginning to smell a rat. But before I knew it they had got me into a flying suit and strapped a parachute on my back, ready to go for a taxi round the airfield ? "Remember" I said to Ian "just a taxi, ON THE GROUND, ROUND THE AIRFIELD." "Of course old boy" he said, as somehow we found ourselves lined up on the main runway, ready for take off. The next thing the laconic phrase 'Tango Alpha, departing zero seven' came over the earphones to be followed by the usual instructor patter of "follow me through". Before I knew it my hands were back on the controls and with Ian in command I was once again feeling the terrific sense of getting airborne.

We climbed out on an easterly heading to circuit height and then turned south onto 180 degrees magnetic, heading for my own village a few miles away. "Thought you might like to have a look at the place where you have been so deeply confined and totally grounded for the last few years" Ian said. It was all coming back to me . The effects of control, the coordination, the throttle setting, the look out, the trim, the command of pitch, roll and yaw. It was true, it had never left me, I could still fly! What an amazing boost to my self confidence and fragile self esteem this pretty smart trick of Ian and Alan's to get me airborne once again was to prove. Over the village I looked down and once again realised the tremendous sense of achievement in overcoming gravity, of the world and of my feelings of depression. This was why I had taken up flying in the first place. To go beyond normal earthly limitations and reach for the stars.

Oh! I have slipped the surly bonds of earth
And danced the skies on laughter–silvered wings;

Having triumphantly soared above my bete noir we headed 360 degrees magnetic for a standard rejoin downwind then "Tango Alpha finals 07" for a text book landing back at Eagle base. My feelings at that moment were indescribable and at that same moment I became aware that the whole squadron team (who I had thought were oblivious to what was going on) were out there lining the dispersal and cheering as we taxied back in. Top Gun and Tom Cruise eat your heart out! I was back.

To misquote Churchill. This was not the end; it was not the beginning of the end; but it was the end of the beginning.

From now on humour was to be my medicine, laughter my food and light heartedness would lift up mine eyes from this muddy vestige to my real self. So in my attempt to be liberated from my own fear and as I cleaned up my act, my family helped to clean up my home. Slowly the all pervading torpor was replaced by creativity and brightness. The indolence was replaced by activity and light. I began to paint with water colours again after a break of many years. I began to read enjoyably and entertain myself with creative writing.

I began by addressing the increased aerodynamic drag force of my mind set and the extra payload of the all up weight of the additional three stones of fat I had taken on board whilst blown off track, and began to exercise in the fresh air and sweet sunshine.

I was always fond of the concept of death or glory; thank God I chose glory! You know before the battle of Blenheim, Marlborough said to his ADC, "Tomorrow we conquer or die!"

Well, this much I have learnt from my own experiences and as my old Philosophy tutor would say, about life, so far- "Never say die"!

So better get on with living then. And a good place to start could be here. Let's see now. What have we learnt from all this?

The truth about depression is:

It is a disease.

It is a real illness.

It IS survivable.

The Spirit in Man is imperishable (not even the deepest depression) can destroy the Spirit.

What depression is not:

It is not imagined.

It is not self indulgence.

It is not forever.

Avoid melancholic tendencies. Avoid self doubt. Avoid self blame. Cultivate awareness, alertness, activity, exercise body and mind. Seek physical, mental and spiritual rest. Eat healthy fresh food. Feed the body, mind and soul. Avoid stress like the plague.

Have a vision but avoid dreaming, circling thoughts, inner conversations, thinking too much. Like Pooh Bear try just 'being' and trust the self knowledge of the senses. Live your life to the fullness of your spirit and be your true self, not some shadow of your thoughts. Reach for the sky, the stars, the universe, the absolute. Go on, touch the face of God.

Oh! I have slipped the surly bonds of earth
And danced the skies on laughter–silvered wings;
Sunwards I have climbed, and joined the tumbling mirth
Of sun–split clouds – and done a hundred things
You have not dreamed of – wheeled and soared and swung
High in the sunlit silence. Hovering there
I've chased the shouting wind along, and flung
My eager craft through footless halls of air.
Up, up the long delirious, burning blue,
I've topped the windswept heights with easy grace
Where never lark, or even eagle flew –
And, while with silent lifting mind I've trod
The high untresspassed sanctity of space,
Put out my hand and touched the face of God.
Pilot Officer Gillespie Magee
No 412 Squadron, RCAF
Killed 11 December 1941

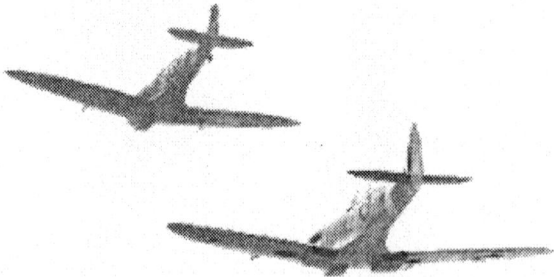

11 HAPPILY EVER AFTER

As the greatest story teller of them all once said: 'All's well that ends well.' And this tale shall not be an exception to that golden rule. This then, perhaps not of my making, but happily of my finding, is just that, a happy ending. It would now seem to be, that all the slings and arrows of outrageous fortune have come to pass, and now have passed. And, notwithstanding all those arrows still in flight, as was always meant to be, now is perfectly well. Since we are told perfect comes from perfect. Take perfect from perfect and the remainder is perfect. Let peace and peace and peace be everywhere.

And so good readers:

Our revels now are ended, or may be not quite. These, our actors, as I foretold are still on stage.

So, what about Kathryn? Careful Kate, cunning Kate, Kate the cursed, as Shakespeare would say? Or JF? What about their relationship? How did they ever come to find themselves in this drama In the first place?

Well this is probably the wrong time to introduce this, but theirs is probably the most extraordinary love affair of all time.

Their star signs could not be more opposed: His Aquarius, hers Scorpio: the horoscope read: 'Bedroom acrobatics will not keep this disparate couple together, let them go their separate ways'. That is until James arrived and the union was blessed with marriage. Starting a young family all over again at such a mature age was quite a shock, but they enjoyed the youthful vitality and the challenge it brought to their lives.

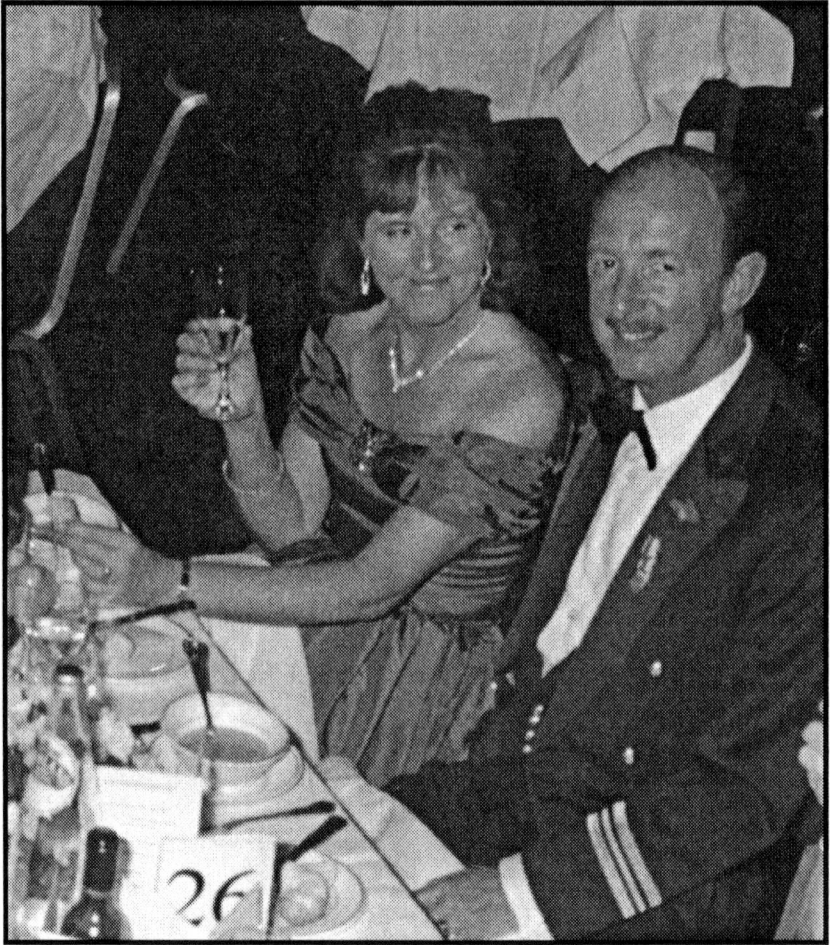

SCORPIO & BIGGLES

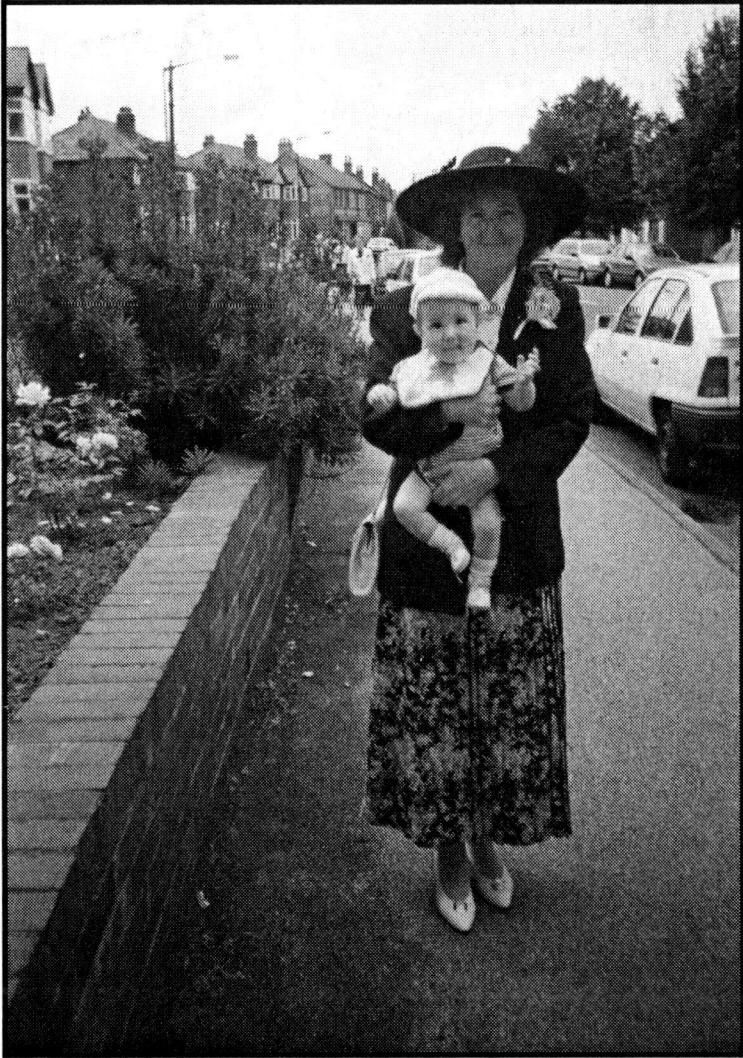

ALONG CAME JAMES!

The adventures of this unlikely liaison were legion. And the stories would fill her book with real life comic tragedies and French Farces. Like the Edgerton Arms and the case of the lost Blue Room. But suffice to know both Kathryn and John have so far survived the vicissitudes of life in some form of loose battle formation.

It was after all, probably the most passionate affair possible. Imagine, The Queen of the Night and Biggles. What aerobatics eh? People would say "Eee, our Elsie, it will never last" that sort of thing. But incredibly it did.

And yet their relationship continued to defy all known laws of gravity. They just enjoyed every other moment of their love affair. The other moment was either the high or low of the swing. He would please her like no other and then they would climb to 40,000 feet. Or displease her and she would cut him dead and run off to tell her close mate, Catherine, who he was to name 'Your delinquent Little Friend' how much she hated him.

(Her wrongly maligned friend, Catherine Roberts, was to go on to become a brilliant proponent of the alternative medicine art of Homeopathy. This amazing, much under valued, science was to help restore me to health after a record double triple heart bypass operation which occurred during the first year of my recovery from the great depression.)

This then was to be the acid test of my recovery. Would such a major trauma return me to the deadly disease in some giant tragic twist in the final melancholic episode of the play? Would I reluctantly have to capitulate to some greater power of fate that decides these things or, by opposing, end there in. Well the jury may still be out, but judging by the occurrence of another major trauma in the form of a mid air collision in which, thank God, all the aircrew, including myself, survived, I would have to say, no.

No thank you Master of Ceremonies or Director of the play. This actor will graciously accept all future challenges, but the lesson of depression, so well courted before in these situations, has now been learnt.

Now where's that Homeopath? I say, about this 'Parkinson's Disease' I have just been diagnosed with?

Well folks, don't miss next weeks exciting episode!

And so now where was I? Oh yes.

These our actors as I foretold you, were all spirits and are melted into air, thin air: and like the baseless fabric of this vision, the cloud-capped towers, the gorgeous palaces, the solemn temples, the great globe itself, yea, all which it inherit' shall dissolve and, like this insubstantial pageant faded, leave not a rack behind. We are such stuff as dreams are made on, and our little life is rounded with a sleep.

BIBLIOGRAPHY

Page	Quote	Author
21	Men Like Machines	John Farron
22	Jonathan Livingston Seagull	Richard Bach
55	The Battle of France.......	Winston Churchill
63	The Self is One......	Eesha Upanishad
65	The friends thou hast......	Shakespeare - Hamlet
78	Full many a glorious morning..	Shakespeare - Sonnet
80	Of a certainty a man who can...	Eesha Upanishad
80	Is Thinking Destroying Your Life	Unknown
94	High Flight (1941)	Pilot Officer Gillespie Magee
99	Our revels now are ended....	Shakespeare - The Tempest

GLOSSARY OF TERMS

Page	Description	
10	Pitot Head	Probe which registers the total oncoming air pressure which after allowance for static atmospheric air pressure is used to register Indicated Air Speed
10	Canberra	Name of Bomber aircraft known as Tactical Strike Reconnaissance One (TSR1) Forerunner to the ill fated TSR2
12	TSR2	As above
16	Met	Abbreviation for Meteorology
16	P of F	Principles of Flight
19	Stall	Point at which the wing ceases to produce lift through disruption of the laminar air flow
19	Spin	Autorotation in spiral dive
20	C of G	Centre of Gravity
20	Altimeter	Gauge for registering height above airfield elevation (QFE) or height above nominal regional pressure level (QNH)
27	Alpha	Angle of attack of oncoming relative air flow to wing
30	Pathos	Deepest depression, sorrow, sadness, pity, suffering, tragedy, misery, grief
30	Flutter	High frequency vibration of wings or control surface
30	Dampening	Reduction of effects of flutter by harmonisation
	STC	Staff Continuation Training

ACKNOWLEDGEMENTS

The Author wishes to acknowledge the help given to him in production of this book by the following people.

Design of front and back cover by Clive Shorrock

Diagram of Causes by Dr Vincent Mainey GP

Forward by Dr Pradip Patel

Review by Group Captain W M N Cross OBE

Eagle and Crown Image – A trade Mark of the Secretary of State for Defence and use with their permission

The Poem - High Flight (1941) by Pilot Officer Gillespie Magee.

Reproduced by kind permission of 'This England' magazine

The du Plessis family of South Africa for the idea of the title "Ice on My Wings"

For unstinting patience and perseverance in the typing of this manuscript - My long suffering, beloved wife Kathryn

Printed in the United Kingdom
by Lightning Source UK Ltd.
119652UK00001B/358-393